T0146124

RIGHT
HEMISPHERE
STROKE

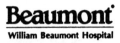
William Beaumont Hospital

William Beaumont Hospital
Speech and Language Pathology Series

MICHAEL I. ROLNICK, PH.D.
Series Editor

RIGHT HEMISPHERE STROKE

A Victim Reflects on Rehabilitative Medicine

Fred K. Johnson

WAYNE STATE UNIVERSITY PRESS DETROIT 1990

94   93   92   91   90   5   4   3   2   1

Library of Congress Cataloging-in-Publication Data
Johnson, Fred K., 1945-
   Right hemisphere stroke : a victim reflects on rehabilitative
medicine / Fred K. Johnson.
      p.   cm.—(William Beaumont Hospital speech and language
pathology series)
      ISBN 0-8143-2172-0 (alk. paper).
      1. Johnson, Fred K., 1945-   —Health.   2. Cerebrovascular
disease—Patients—United States—Biography.   3. Cerebrovascular
disease—Patients—Rehabilitation.   I. Title.   II. Series.
RC388.5.J616   1990
362.1'9681—dc20   89-70612
                                                              CIP

The author has donated the original long-hand manuscript of this book and
subsequent typed revisions to the University of Texas, where they are housed
in the Barker Texas History Center. Wayne State University Press has donated
the proofs and copies of the editorial correspondence to the Center.

With a large measure of respect and affection this book is dedicated to Lynne Hayes, Ph.D., a most gifted and compassionate speech-language pathologist. Lynne realized a right-hemisphere stroke victim would benefit from her gentle art. When I came to her I could not write or read. She helped me to find the path back.

Indeed, the entire history of neurology and neuropsychology can be seen as the investigation of the left hemisphere.

Oliver Sacks, M.D.

Contents

Foreword

My thirty years of practice has brought me into contact with hundreds of strokes in my role as clinician and clinical investigator, and I have been impressed by the infinite variety of presentation and prognosis that I have seen. No two strokes are identical. On the surface they may seem to have this appearance — every physician knows that a right hemisphere stroke causes left-sided weakness — but, unfortunately, the majority of medical professionals believe this stereotype and do not spend time to search beneath the surface and discover how the stroke has affected the patient as a whole person. There are many reasons for this nihilistic attitude, including the lack of inclination to spend the necessary time to study one individual and the persistence of the outrageous dogma that "there is not much you can do for a stroke anyway." This attitude is too common, and the minority who are truly dedicated to the full rehabilitation of the stroke victim conduct a never-ending struggle to educate and change beliefs.

One need only compare the therapy and rehabilitation of the patient with a heart attack to the benign approach or neglect of the patient with a "brain attack," for that is the exact nature of a stroke. Indeed, the name may be of vital importance in the development of attitude in the case of a stroke.

It is imperative, then, that the treatment of the stroke victim be based on an intelligent approach to the problem with a realistic optimism — that much can be done. This book by Fred K. Johnson illustrates this very well, and I congratulate him on the production of a work which should be read by all medical students, students of rehabilitation, and practicing health professionals. It is clear from the first chapter that no two strokes are alike, that each patient should be thoroughly evaluated to identify the many deficits which accompany the stroke, and that there should be adequate communication and an ongoing educational program for the various health personnel engaged in stroke rehabilitation.

Fred Johnson's case illustrates the complexity of a stroke. He shows us that there is no such thing as a right hemisphere or left hemisphere stroke since he suffered so many deficits which are usually thought to be left hemisphere functions following the right carotid occlusion. In other words, although the author does not so state, a stroke affects the brain as a whole, and patients should be treated for brain dysfunction, not hemisphere deficits.

Johnson's story also illustrates the need for better communication with the patient. The physician does not emerge unscathed: there is a noticeable lack of contact with the patient. Every patient suffering from a first stroke should be told that he or she will walk again. This is a reasonable assumption and a remarkable morale booster for the patient and the family. Similarly, the rehabilitation of a stroke patient is a complex problem which should be discussed openly. This was not done in Johnson's case, where information was gathered in a fragmented fashion—almost serendipitously. The problems present or anticipated in many other diseases are freely discussed with patients and family (no surgeon would remove a brain tumor without a preliminary discussion of the procedure, risks, and outcome with the patient and family), but the attitude towards stroke includes a hidden agenda, as though there is something shameful in acknowledging the presence of this complex problem.

We are approaching the time when more effective treatment will be available for the stroke victim in the acute phase and in rehabilitation. This will be facilitated by bringing the subject out of the closet and discussing its many facets. Fred Johnson's story is an excellent opening salvo. We need his insight and his determination, and we are fortunate that he continues to work for the stroke victim and will hopefully do so for years to come.

John Gilroy, M.D., P.C., FRCP (CAN) FACP
Chairman of Neurology, William Beaumont
Hospital, Royal Oak, MI
Clinical Professor of Neurology, Wayne State
University

Introduction

The original title of this volume was *God Could Have Written Me a Letter*. That thought reflects the feelings of many stroke victims. The phrase "right hemisphere" was placed in the title to better describe what this book entails. It is the story of a right-hemisphere stroke victim's ordeal. As the epigraph to this book implies, the right hemisphere has often been overlooked. Because of this oversight, there is a lack of understanding as to what to expect when the right hemisphere of the brain is damaged. Hopefully, this book will contribute needed knowledge to this area. However, I suspect that there is more overlap between the right hemisphere and the left in function than is generally thought.

Based upon conversations with my doctors and with other right-hemisphere stroke victims, I exhibited many of the traits typical of right-hemisphere stroke victims. Yet it should not be thought that all right-hemisphere stroke victims will suffer through the same experiences I did. However, both left- and right-hemisphere stroke victims may suffer the same horrors and experiences I did.

The difficulty in trying to describe the quintessential right-hemisphere stroke victim is that there are no typical strokes. Certainly no two strokes are alike. The fact that no strokes are alike should be remembered before demanding that a loved one receive the same therapy that worked for Fred Johnson in his book. Although our strokes may seem similar, they are in fact different.

The lack of a thorough understanding of the overall effects of right-hemisphere damage should not be used as an excuse for shying away from rehabilitative treatment. The medical management of right- and left-hemisphere stroke victims is much the same. There is a growing awareness that right-hemisphere stroke

1

victims should receive evaluation for speech, language, and cognitive therapy. This is a decided change for the better.

Regrettably, the pressure of publication deadlines did not allow the time to secure the proper authorizations to use the real names of the hospitals and many doctors and therapists who helped me. Helen Wulf's work with *A Stroke of Luck* is recognized nationally. Josephine Simonson is known for her interest in aphasiology. Thus, their real names are used. So that the dedication to this book may be better understood, I have used Lynne Hayes's real name. Although most of the names have been changed, the story is a true one. My memory is fair—that in itself should simplify the telling of my tale. But many stroke stories follow a simple pattern: the hospital and the return from the hospital to pick up the pieces—a simple two-stage story.

The hospital phase is full of drama. Will the patient live? Will he walk? How will the bills be paid? During this stage of uncertainty, there is a sense of suspense, which helps to move my story along. By the time of the patient's release from the hospital, many of the questions have been answered. The focus of the story shifts to how the family copes. It is at this stage that one sees the stroke as the family affair it truly is.

Fortunately in my story, the wolf was not at the door, so there was little one could do to maintain the tension and suspense of the first stage of my story in the second stage. The two or three years of post-stroke life I write about are true—not glamorous but true.

At this point a natural tension can arise between an editor and an author. The editor may cry, "The story falls apart in the middle. Add some pizzazz to it." The writer replies, "My life *fell* apart in the middle. All I can do is tell it the way it happened." I'm pleased that the editors at Wayne State University Press adopted the reasonable attitude of keeping me on a tight rein, but allowing me to tell my story as it happened.

A few editors might have felt uneasy with some of the spiritual references which crop up in my story. Yet these spiritual experiences may be common for certain people who have suffered many types of head injuries. In keeping with the secular sophistication of the day, it would have been tempting for the editor to sweep all spiritual references under the carpet. Again, these spiritual episodes can be common in head injuries. I know both left- and right-hemisphere stroke victims who have indeed experienced them.

It is far from clear if these religious delusions are a function of the damaged right hemisphere of the brain (or, as I suspect, trauma in general). It is only by retaining references to them that future clinicians will be better able to evaluate if this is truly a right-hemisphere manifestation. Again, the editors are to be commended for retaining material that will allow such future evaluations of this intriguing area.

I'm vain enough to hope you have selected this book for its literary merits. If you turned to this book because a loved one had a stroke and you are seeking answers, have courage. If they lived long enough for you to have found this book, they have crossed the first hurdle: they lived—no small thing. It is far too easy to lose hope and question when they will regain consciousness, or talk, or walk. Rather than demanding "when," remember that they have already taken the first step. They chose to live. Courage!

God Could Have Written Me a Letter

At this moment I would like to ignore the religious implications of the title of this chapter. I am no modern-day Job. In the proper place, I will speak of some of the religious fantasies or illusions that accompanied my stroke. This volume is basically a factual account of my actions and reactions in trying to adjust to the new world I encountered after I suffered a stroke, which paralyzed my left side.

In the aftermath of my stroke, there have been many changes in my life-style—no more candy bars, booze, or cigarettes; the fast women and slow horses are all gone. Their replacements are extra-iron vitamin tablets and church on Sunday. What a transformation! It would make any wife proud. I have embraced the good life, yet I think the stroke was a heavy price to pay to get on the straight and narrow. All in all, I would have preferred that God had written me a letter—a stroke struck me as being a little heavy-handed.

The day of my stroke (Memorial Day, 1981) started off as a perfectly ordinary day. There were no precursors of doom that morning. My wife, Judy, gave me a perfunctory good-bye kiss as she left for work. My son was already up watching the TV cartoons. I was pretending to quit smoking at the time, but a craving for nicotine and my dislike of the din of the cartoons motivated me to roll out of bed, get dressed, and stretch out on the recliner on the back porch. The porch was screened in. I lit up. The smoke would not linger; the boy would not see. The day looked to be ordinary; if not for the stroke, it would have been.

For the less medically inclined, a stroke is the stoppage of the flow of blood to the brain. At first that does not sound too bad, for ours is the age of technocrats in which satellites repair themselves. Unfortunately, the brain has not benefited from this evolution of technology. When the brain is without blood, parts of it die. For a moment, let's key in on the word "die." It is too easy to get lost or confused in the medical jargon of left or right hemispheres when there are only two kinds of strokes, those that kill you and those that don't. Needless to say, mine was of the latter kind.

The Porch

As I said, the day was ordinary. I was on a recliner on my back porch smoking a cigarette and listening to life awakening as the Florida sun rose. The passage from that tranquil time to my stroke was rather routine; there were no bolts of lightning or bursts of fire. I dropped my pack of cigarettes and while reaching to retrieve them, I fell unceremoniously onto the concrete patio. After a while, I realized that I could not get up; my left arm and leg were not moving. That did not strike me as being odd at the time. I knew it was not right, but I did not think it was wrong since there was no pain or anything else to indicate anything violently wrong with my head or body.

After a while, I concluded that it was uncomfortable lying on the concrete, so I called to my son, Sam, to bring me a pillow. I continued to grope for my package of cigarettes. With the pillow tucked under my head, I calmly awaited events.

I again called Sam to help me get up; I wanted to lie down on the couch and take a real nap. Sam came and tried to help me to my feet. Half standing, we crashed through my wife's array of flower pots. I found myself on the floor again, this time in pain from a scraped knee.

I then realized that Sam would not be able to help me get up; I asked him to get the neighbor to help. The neighbor, who was a policeman and might have recognized what was going on, was on duty. Sam got our other neighbor, the accountant, who most likely thought I was drunk and did not give my physical condition a thought while dragging me to the bedroom. Sam called my wife, Judy. She came home and called the ambulance. I never did find the pack of cigarettes.

Rather than being a sleek red hearse-type ambulance, mine was a squared-off emergency vehicle that looked rather like an ice-cream truck. The paramedics continually asked me if I had a headache or if I had hit my head in the fall. I replied, "NO," and tried to point out that my arm and leg were paralyzed. This now struck me as serious.

Medical Treatment

My most vivid memory of the hospital emergency room is that my doctor manhandled me to spread me across a desk top to do a spinal tap. I'm six feet tall and weigh 180 pounds, so it was not easy to drape me across a desk. Aside from a strong desire to sleep, I have few other memories of the emergency room. Six months later, I was to recall that I felt the chill of death and heard the wing beats of the Angel of Death.

As a child, I had a fondness for the poems of Joyce Kilmer, especially for "Rouge Bouquet" and its haunting litany of the Angels of Death led by St. Michael in an angelic salute: "St. Michael's soward darts through the air and touches the aureole of his hair." It may well be that the memory of Kilmer's verse acted to stimulate my mind to imagine that I heard the wing beats of the Angel of Death.

Be that as it may, I did feel the presence of death. But by and by, it was judged that I was stable, so I was taken to a standard hospital room. Hell, things should have been looking up: I got out of the emergency room in one piece. But my left leg and arm were paralyzed, and, although I did not realize it, a great deal of my mental faculties were impaired. In short, I was in poor shape. But it beats the hell out of dying!

The current medical wisdom is to begin therapy as soon as possible after the stroke. Thus, I was hardly out of intensive care before I was poked and prodded in the rehabilitation process. This rehabilitation process continued for nearly a year, day after day. I even had homework on the weekends. There is no rest for the weary in rehabilitation land.

It has been a long haul, and right from the beginning of this odyssey I had doctor problems. I had been to my doctor a week before the stroke complaining of a transient numbness in my left arm. He recommended that I stop taking medicine for my high blood pressure. Needless to say, I was left without a great deal of faith in that doctor.

Then a host of outside medical experts came in. After a while, I felt like the fatted calf ready for the slaughter. Every doctor in Dade County seemed to review my case, but I never found out what they concluded. With all of the neurologists, physiatrists, and plumbers who saw me, you would think there would be someone who would tell me what was going on.

Prior to my stroke I was the director of labor relations for a large manufacturing conglomerate, and I would negotiate contracts with unions across the country. Union contract negotiations are often a bluff built upon a well-planned strategy. You have an idea of what you are going to do and how things will turn out. There are no guarantees, but you develop a feeling for how things will end up. It comes down to the old adage, "You pay your nickel and you take your chances," based on your experience and best judgment. That is the world I came from, where answers were tough but there *were* answers.

But all the specialists on my case seemed unable or unwilling to give me a straight answer to my question, "Will I ever walk again?" They would hunch up and look busy and say, "Work hard."

When I would not be submissive and would ask them to make an educated guess, the specialists would be all the more evasive. This caused me to feel that the doctors were not telling me the whole truth. I was accustomed to making educated guesses. (Would the union strike if I did not give them a holiday?) I did not consider it unreasonable to ask my doctors for an educated prediction. Given these circumstances, it is not uncommon for stroke victims to become paranoid. It began to seem reasonable to *me* to become paranoid.

My hospital room was on a floor with a number of other stroke patients. There was a physical therapy gym on the same floor as well as a common eating area. I was not in any kind of rehabilitation center, though; I was still in an acute-care hospital area. I was put into acute care because the cause of my stroke was unknown. Thus, a second stroke might be in the wings. As a result, a delicate balance had to be maintained. It is tempting to think that you may as well be comfortable while you are waiting to see how things turn out. But the therapists do not want such a mamby pamby patient! Well, consider how such a patient might feel. He is hurt, confused, and afraid. No one tells him the score. Such a patient may want to rest and lick his wounds. But there is no rest. The morning after my stroke, my therapy began.

The ward nurses were going to teach me how to dress. They were not occupational therapists, but floor nurses—and they were going to teach me at the start of the day when they were the most rushed. This is a clear example of what I was to experience all too much. Stroke patients can be stomped, spindled, and pushed into any crevice of the hospital routine; it is so easy to make us bend to the system. We cannot walk out and oftentimes we cannot speak to complain. If we could, who would listen? It is well known that stroke patients are often paranoid. Since the system seems to have helped me, I will curb my bitter outbursts for the moment. But before we resume with the floor nurses teaching me to dress, it is well to consider the use of the word "forget" with stroke patients.

"Forget," like charity, covers a multitude of sins. The patient's problems come about because he forgets. It is a nice, soft verb. We all forget things. If we forget to pick up the laundry, we can always go back to the cleaners. No big deal. It is so much nicer to say "forget" in lieu of "his brain is dead." "Forget" is a gentle verb and carries an implied hope of remembering.

In keeping with this optimistic outlook, one might say that I forgot how to read a clock or that my left arm forgot how to work. Given my labor relations background, I always said my arm was on a wildcat strike. I had not forgotten how to dress, but I did have difficulty dressing for a number of reasons. The obvious reason was that my left arm was not working. The less obvious one involved some vision difficulties to be discussed later. Whatever the causes of the problem, I was prodded into learning to dress, and I resisted.

Why would I resist? Didn't I want to get well? The principal problem with my dressing was that my left arm was on strike. Aside from not being able to pull up my underwear, it was a bitch to thread my dead-weight arm into a shirt sleeve. There were ways to overcome these problems. Why not adapt to them? At the time it seemed to me that to learn new dressing techniques was to admit and outwardly affirm that my left arm was going to be paralyzed forever. That was throwing in the towel too early. Didn't they know that winners never quit and quitters never win? I didn't want to give up on the arm so easily. Looking back now, these arguments seem pale and empty. However, at the time, they appeared quite persuasive and cogent.

In therapy, the phrase "getting well" is not synonymous with the concept of being healed or made whole. Getting well is learning how to cope—how to be independent. That seems to be a noble sentiment, but I always thought it was the first step to becoming an invalid!

I didn't want to learn to be an invalid; I did not want to live in a wheelchair or learn to compensate for my arm. I wanted to be healed. That is why I was in the hospital, or so I thought. And, of course, I wanted to sleep and be left alone, to let my body heal itself since no one else could heal me.

I saw a number of aphasic patients who seemed to have the same resistance to therapy that I had. To repeat the point, the resistance to a program of therapy for a given deficit does not mean that one denies the deficit. To resist the therapy is not to deny the problem. As Elisabeth Kübler-Ross's book *On Death and Dying* gains greater acceptance, there is a danger of taking her stages of denial and applying them out of context when dealing with stroke patients. I felt an unrelenting pressure to admit that I was very sick throughout my hospital confinement. There was a pressure to submit and throw myself on the nurses' desk and ask for mercy.

Fortunately, I had the will to resist. Although I do not want to belabor the point, I think it *is* important to start therapy early even if the patient is not ready to slide meekly under the thumb of the stroke team. I was in a delicate balance. I needed therapy, but my will to resist was strong; the stroke had not killed it. We will do well to remember that Nietzsche taught that the will to resist is a key to being a superman.

Before things get entirely out of hand, we need to stop and think in terms of that Saturday afternoon matinee movie we all saw when we were younger. You will recall the line in the western when the hero tells the stranger, "I want my horses tame, not broken." Certainly there is a need to tame headstrong patients, but not to break them. Although some stroke patients never get with it, I doubt that you would need even a special routine to tame the stroke patient. The workings of the hospital will tame the patient in spite of himself.

Time was not healing me, it just allowed me a chance to be buffeted around in the normal hospital routine, a process that would take off my rough edges. What passed for routine was in reality the stripping away of individuality; my life was reduced to getting up and going to therapy.

In former days when I sat at bargaining tables, I would laugh and tell union officials that I was flexible. However, I was very regimented. There was always another meeting or a plane to catch. I would go about bringing order to a world of chaos. Please do not conclude that I was overly fastidious or that I always plowed straight furrows. I was orderly, but I never suffered from a compulsion to be neat. However, like many stroke victims I had disorientation problems.

Disorientation merits a large digression because it is one of the factors that can tame a patient. Time disorientation is more than just forgetting how to read clocks. (Notice how soft and forgiving is the sound of the verb "forget.")

My time disorientation had nothing to do with the reading of clocks. I lost sense of my place in time and was adrift. The failure of my senses to mark (or perhaps the word is "remember") the passage of time left me without references. My feeling of being adrift is perhaps best explained by my wife's account of a night of terror when I thought I had lost my family because I had lost my sense of time. My wife's account follows:

> At 2:00 in the afternoon, I told you I was going to pick up Sam at school and that we were going to the movies. You went to sleep. At 7:00 that evening, you woke up and thought it was 7:00 in the morning. You thought you had slept straight through the afternoon, evening, and night and that we had not come to see you after the movie. You picked up the phone and called home, and there was no answer. We were still at the movies. You jumped to the conclusion that something terrible had happened to us, because we should have been home having breakfast if it was really 7:00 in the morning, as you thought.
>
> A half-hour later at 7:30, Sam and I arrived at the hospital. It took me an hour to convince you that only five hours had passed, not twelve.

That half hour was one of real terror for me. Judy's story is just too simple. There *must* have been an evening meal to wake me up and then another nap that merged into what I thought was the next day.

If you are uncharitable, you might conclude that the above story reinforces the point that stroke patients are paranoid. Given Miami's history of drug and race warfare, it is reasonable to be fearful if you have lost track of your wife and family. To reiterate the point, my disorientation affected my relationship with the outside world.

Disorientation

The time disorientation was also a hindrance to my re-employment possibilities. I kept in touch with my employer by telephone, and there were many times when I would call my boss on a Friday and before hanging up say that I would call him again the next day. Each time he reminded me that the next day was a nonworking Saturday, I felt foolish and feared that by demonstrating my weakness I was endangering my job.

When I asked my doctor about this loss of orientation he would merely say that it is common for hospital patients to lose track of which day it was. I did not feel that putting a calendar on the wall would have been a big help. My wife favors a digital clock that has the date and day on it. I never felt a compulsion to know the date, but I did like to know the month.

My mother sent me a Timex LCD quartz battery-powered watch that shows the month, day, date, and time; I again had command over time. With the watch safely on my wrist, was I cured? That question has more substance than is immediately apparent. Throughout my recovery, I always sought a magic, simple cure, such as a watch. The magic I coveted for my left arm was the electrical wiring of the bionic man. For my eyes and my reading problems, some glasses would help me get the proper focus.

That was my simple wish list. However, rather than having these wishes granted by magic, I brought them to the altar of technology. Perhaps that is the altar of a false god—the magic is within. Throughout the therapy process I dreamed of magic and miracles. Of course, one cannot dream all of the time, and I occasionally reflected with fear and trembling upon some of my problems of which I was aware, but which remained vague and elusive.

When one has problems of time disorientation, it is possible to have problems with locations and spatial relationships. That, in short, means you can get lost in a bathtub. And I did.

I still bitterly rage that no one saw fit to tell me that I might have these problems. It is not that we were on the cutting edge of medical science: the facts are well known. Knowledge about time and spatial disorientation is not confined to the great research hospitals. Everyone knew about left- or right-hemisphere strokes, but I was the last to learn what medical science knew about some of my problems. Why hide these problems under a basket? Why should stroke victims write books like this one to provide information? Because the practitioners will not share the information with the patients. The royalties are not that great and no reason in themselves to motivate a project like this.

Patient reader, you have the right to demand, "Fred, stop this diatribe and tell us more about your secret problem of spatial disorientation." All right. I felt as though I was in the same position as so many of the husbands in those unbearable jokes about unfaithful wives. My problem wasn't a secret; it's just that I didn't know.

The thing I didn't know was that stroke victims often (usually) have problems with their sense of direction. I would get lost in the hallway. To my credit, it should be noted that the hallway had a few dog-leg turns. To get to physical therapy and the dining area, I would have to take a left turn and I exited my room and follow the dog-log turns. To get back to my room, I would also have to make a left when I departed from therapy. On the face of it, it seemed simple enough: everything is down the hall. But there is many a slip betwixt the cup and the lip.

Oftentimes I would forget which way to turn to go to therapy. Meals were no great problem, you just went with the herd; however, to return was a real chore. If I went to the right when I was leaving therapy (the wrong direction), I would be on a seemingly endless corridor with no hope of redemption. I would, however, push on, looking for the room of a girl from New York, which inexplicably had a recliner in it. This was one of my trail markers to let me know that I had taken the correct path back to my room.

I had the habit of staring into people's rooms as I wheeled by, a potentially embarrassing practice, but after a while you can do it with some aplomb. Those of you less willing to stare into the hospital rooms of sick folks might ask, "Fred, why not just read the signs?" Although I stand a good, honest six feet tall, in a wheelchair I'm not that tall and I missed a lot of signs.

I laughed at the painted lines on the floor. So you want me

to bend forward in a wheelchair when I have no balance? I could pivot over and rotate like a human ferris wheel. Signs are only useful if you see them. I was still having trouble adjusting to looking to the right and to the left. And, of course, signs are only helpful if you know where you are going. The signs never read, "This way to Fred's room." To understand "Rooms 2000-3000" required more math or more organizational sense than I possessed.

Whenever my wife visited me and found my room empty, she would ask at the nurses' station where I was. The invariable answer was a mocking, "You know how Fred is, he's probably lost in the halls." I will leave to your imagination what type of strain that could cause to a marriage already in disarray.

If I were to say to anyone that my nurses were not the descendants of Florence Nightingale, there would be an instant rejoinder of, "Fred, all patients say that about rehab nurses." However, I will not be dissuaded from my opinions.

In the beginning, since the nurses would not answer my call button at night, my urinal tended to overflow. My wife had to sneak into the hospital in the morning before wake-up time with rags to clean me up. I still weep when I recall that my wife had to sneak in with rags. Her conduct was immediately labeled as "disruptive of hospital routine."

The controls to raise or lower my bed were in a small hand control connected by a heavy cord to the electric motor beneath my bed. I never quite mastered this hand control. When I wanted to raise the head of the bed, I would press a button. If the foot of the bed declined, I would stop and shift to another button. It seems that I could not remember which button I had already pressed, so my scientific method of pressing buttons would not work.

One afternoon, I had managed to break the great rule about not being in bed during the day. My back hurt, and I wanted to raise the head of the bed, so I pressed a button. The foot of the bed went down with the shrill engine sound you associate with an engine on its last legs. My frustrations increased as I continued to fail in selecting the correct hand-control button.

At that time, my nurse, Martha, strolled in. I asked her if she could please make my bed go up. In an instant her posture was ramrod straight as she hissed, "Johnson, I ain't no maid. I made that bed up this morning. I ain't making it up again!"

The critical reader might wonder, "Fred, did you ever like people? Were you always a stick in the mud?"

This is a fair question, with a complex answer. Prior to my stroke, I never really cared for people very much. After the stroke,

I was a warmer, more affable person, despite my experiences with some nurses. This change was not a gradual evolution in my personality. It was a radical transformation, a quantum jump that I was not aware of at first. In concert with the time disorientation and the trouble with spatial relationships, a stroke victim may experience personality changes. As you might expect, I was not told that such changes were likely to occur. No doubt a doctor might argue that there is no need to concern the poor patient; he or she has enough problems without being concerned about things which may never happen. That answer seems sound, but it leaves the patient to wonder if he is going mad.

Lusting-After

Again, I would stress that the changes in my personality were radical shifts. There was no Dr. Jekyll and Mr. Hyde effect with a vacillation from one personality to the other; I just came up as a warmer, more agreeable person. Months later, I was to describe this evolution as a reincarnation.

In addition to the desirable changes noted above, I lost some of my inhibitions. The rusty chains of a Catholic childhood were broken and scraped. The rigid stone wall of a character molded in the South developed fissures. The man from the home office was without a portfolio: "Things fell apart, the center would not hold."

I found real pleasure in glancing down the blouses of young women, at the creamy softness. Ah, the sights of a thousand nights! I did not become a dirty old man or a masher, I was just reintroduced to the pleasure of lusting-after, which I had lost somewhere along the way. The stroke had sliced through that part of my brain where my inhibitions were centered. Certainly no great loss; it is only with the greatest restraint that I avoid speaking of "gold and silver linings."

One might think, "Fred, it *is* unfortunate that you found this rekindled flame, yet you hated all of your nurses." Never did I say that I hated nurses. As we shall see later on, I was very fond of those at a different hospital.

But I did suddenly become enamored of beautiful speech pathologists. If I made the categorical statement that all speech pathologists are beautiful women, one might object and ask, "Fred, how large is the sample on which you base this broad generalization?"

I worked with three speech pathologists in two states and

have had the pleasure of speaking at three of their large conventions. My credentials now firmly established, I would like to return to my point. Speech pathologists *do* tend to be beautiful women. This is said with the reservations implied when one says nurses tend to be women. Enough! There must be a point to all this and, indeed, there is.

While I was having these personality changes, I worked with a beautiful speech pathologist. I was not aphasic, but I thought my speech had been affected by the stroke. It seemed to me that I stuttered or slurred my words. I use the word "seems" because everyone told me how well I spoke; no one was willing to admit to me that my speech was impaired. The fact that everyone refused to admit the obvious did not give me much solace. I thought my father handled the question of my speech rather well. He said that I spoke more deliberately, and he thought that to be an improvement. Since he was the only one who would admit there was a change, I believed him. Before that, though, I was very concerned about my speech. Thus, I began working with a speech pathologist.

The fact that she was beautiful helped diminish my immediate reaction of "let's wait a few days and hope it goes away." The fact is that I wanted my old powers back. Up to that time, I had made my living by being persuasive. My identity, the focus of my being, was grounded in my ability to speak well. I was not about to accept the idea of life in a wheelchair, but wheelchair or not, if I could get to the bargaining table I could be persuasive. I was still a silver-tongued devil, even though a slur or stutter tarnished the silver a bit.

Although I have no frame of reference, I believe that my speech exercises were normal. A lot of effort was devoted to pronouncing Kaputaka, Nantucket, and other assorted tongue twisters, and I was advised to chew gum as homework. The chewing gum brought Demosthenes to mind, and I joked about deducting the cost of the gum from my taxes (I didn't, but it *should* be deductible). Although perhaps whimsical, the chewing of the gum *did* have a positive effect.

One of the more attractive things about my speech pathologist was that she wore real clothes, dresses and nylons, not the universal jeans and bleached white lab coat that seemed the required dress of most of the people I worked with. My speech pathologist literally brought color into my life.

After a few days of being dazzled by my clinician, I decided that we needed to do some different speech exercises. One week of pronouncing Kaputaka and Nantucket will do anyone in. She was not *that* beautiful. So I asked for some practice on how to deal with the telephone.

It seemed that mixed in with some of the personality changes I was experiencing I was losing my aggressiveness and assertiveness. I would shiver and quake when I dialed the switchboard operator on the phone. My voice had a crying moan that was related to my loss of aggressiveness. I never considered that this was anything other than a straightforward speech problem. So I asked for therapy, and we played a few telephone games—a welcome diversion from Kaputaka.

One morning, when I finished physical therapy early (I didn't finish early; they were just done with me early), I wheeled into my speech pathologist's office. No chance of getting lost this time: her office was directly across the hall. There was a yellow pad and pencil lying innocently on her desk. I decided to try writing a few sentences. My handwriting was illegible. I did not maintain margins, and I left letters out of my words. The whole thing was just a shade shy of disaster. Of course, my clinician came in wearing a smashing suede outfit and asked me to read the mess I had written. She pointed to the individual pencil scribbles while I translated. I fumbled through as best I could. I was not about to be shamed in front of that beautiful woman that day. I knew she was kind, but there had to be a way to save face. I fell back on my silver tongue. I told her a rambling story:

> My secretary at work is the only person who can read my writing. You want me to spell? I couldn't spell before the stroke. That kind of reminds me of the man who broke his finger and asked the doctor if he would be able to play the piano. The doctor replied, "Sure." The man said, "That's funny. I couldn't play it before." I'll tell you an apocalyptical story, God's honest truth. When I was in the ninth grade, Mrs. Jason, my English teacher, rebuked me in front of the entire class, saying, "Fred, if you don't learn to spell, no company will ever hire you." I immediately replied that if I could write, the company would hire someone who would spell for me.

It is of no consequence that my objections had a ring of truth to them. I was just being my charming, evasive self. When discussing getting dressed in the morning, I stated that to resist therapy was not to deny the problem. My dodging of the issue of my writing, however, may have been a denial of the problem. I think I was just skirting the issue. I certainly did not want to know that my ability to write a coherent, legible paragraph was impaired.

Although I was not ready or able at the time to confront my writing problem, there were other "mental" problems cropping up that I could not ignore. My father said in his colorful Georgian manner that I had more problems than I could say grace over.

Reading

It seemed that I could not read. Yes, I used "seemed" again, and so that sentence tends to beg the question as to whether I could read or could not read. The answer is somewhat enigmatic. It seemed to me that I could and then again that I could not. My reading ability kind of came and went.

Perhaps you live in an either-or world, where the answer to the question of whether you can read demands a concrete yes or no. After the stroke, I was destined to leave that fine black and white world and enter a gray universe where things were not so clear. Many things were obscured in a cloud of smoke where black merged into gray. Unfortunately, the answer to the question of whether my left arm would or would not work remained a resounding, concrete "NO!" The answer to the question of whether I could read was only a weak "no."

A few weeks after I had entered the hospital, my wife brought me a novelette to read, *The Triumph of Evil* by Paul Kavanaugh. Although not well known, this is a fine little book that received good reviews. I had read it many times prior to the stroke; it had the proper balance of sex and violence to draw me back to it again and again.

As I tried to read the book in bed, I would look at the top of the first page and nod off to sleep. By the time I finally reached the bottom of the first page, I had forgotten what I had read. When I stopped napping, I would turn the page. Since I had read the book a number of times, I knew what was going on. I repeated the pattern of nodding off and turning pages; after a bit, I realized that I was not reading, but just turning pages. I was somewhat lethargic about this and concluded it was more important to take a nap.

It was not my reading material that was putting me to sleep;

for the first time in my life, reading was difficult. When I would see an isolated word, I could understand it. It was when the words were strung together in a sentence that I had trouble. As I have come to understand it, the problem was grounded in my short-term memory and in my propensity to quit at the first difficulty. Whenever I would try to read, I would often start at the top of the page and re-read the material I had just finished. Since my memory was not working well, I would not notice that I was reading the same passage over and over again. As I continued, a sense of lassitude would set in, heightened by the fact that I had read the book previously and knew what was going to happen.

I'm not an academician and do not know how to describe what I was doing. I could call it reading without comprehension, but to me that is a contradiction since to me reading has always implied comprehension. (Of course, I never had to read too much of my own material.) As with most of my problems, the doctor was calm when I talked to him about it. He would point to the signs and ask me to read the word. When I would say the word, the doctor, after dutifully patting my shoulder, would say, "See, Fred, you can read."

My wife, an excellent improviser, started to sneak into my room with a copy of the large-print *Reader's Digest*. She would crawl into bed with me, open the magazine, and start pointing out the words one at a time. I would then say the word out loud. My comprehension of paragraphs, however, was still lacking.

Judy left me a few books on the nightstand, but my interest was not aroused. My reading remained limited to signs in the hospital and the *Daily Shopper* I would find in the waiting rooms. Signs in hospitals do not make pleasant reading material. After I realized that "soiled laundry" did not refer to the gardener's coveralls, I concluded that perhaps it was for the better that I could not yet read signs well. Articles in the *Daily Shopper* were not much better. One issue had an article on the influence of the second international conference on labor Zionism.

I would not want to accuse any of my therapists of giving me false hopes; if anything, they could be indicted for not giving me any hope. Perhaps misunderstanding a therapist's explanation, I began to think my reading problems came about because the muscles that rotated my eyes were impaired, and all I would need were some glasses to retrain the muscles—a manageable problem with a reasonable solution.

Knowing then that the eye problem would work out, it just became a matter of grin and bear it. Since my reading ability seemed to fade in and out as a function of the quality of the material to be read, I would laugh and say that God was giving me editorial control. No signs about soiled laundry. No *Daily Shopper* with its second internationals. It wasn't all bad. I just could not read junk anymore. I could laugh about this editing of my reading material because I was sure that with the proper glasses I would be made whole. However, I did notice that whenever I talked to my therapists about glasses, they would give me a thousand-yard stare.

Since in all probability she did not exist, I could not find the therapist who had told me about the glasses. I vainly looked for her to get more reassurances and to ask, "Why not get the glasses now?" Things were serious. It is all right to make jokes about not reading junk, but to be unable to read—that is to be a barbarian. I needed a glimmer of hope, so I talked to the unit physiatrist (yes, "physiatrist," not "psychiatrist"; a physiatrist specializes in physical medicine and rehabilitation) when I met him in the hallway. He bit his wrist so that his watch was under his nose. This was his shorthand method of showing me that he was busy. Nevertheless, he managed to say, with his wrist still in his mouth, "Fred, the muscles that move your eyes are dead. They may get better; they may not. You must wait and see if there is any return. Right now, accept that you will never read again; if you do, so much the better."

I began to curse and cry. The doctor asked the nurse to restrain me. She got a bed sheet and tied me to the wheelchair. I was a prisoner in an endless hospital corridor in front of Mr. Jackson's room. Jackson was a seventy-year-old black man who had had a stroke when the medical profession did not know how to handle rehabilitation too well. Mr. Jackson's affected arm was strapped to his body for years; this was the accepted treatment for a distended shoulder. In order to unfreeze the shoulder joint, the therapists would raise his arm. They were doing that while I was outside his room. Jackson's shouts of pain were coupled with a stream of profanity a Billie Styron would have marveled at.

Being tied to my wheelchair with the brakes set, I could not wheel out of the flow of Jackson's pain. I joined in his cursing, but my cursing was for those who said I would never again be able to read. There were not only doctors to be damned, there was fate, too. Certainly it was not written on stone tablets that I was to be left with no dignity, that I could not read.

At that moment, my wife, who had come to visit me, found me in the hallway. After wheeling me back to my room, untying the bed sheet, and wiping some tears from my eyes, she asked softly, "Fred, what is the matter?" I tearfully replied, "The doctor said that I might never read again. No one will give me a straight answer, honey. You talk to these people, you must know. Please tell me. Damn it, I'm man enough to take it, please tell me the truth."

I cursed Judy for the next five minutes for withholding the truth from me. When I surpassed her limit, she bent over me and told me that she loved me, then she left softly. She located a psychiatrist who had been working with me. Then the pair descended upon me.

Judy wheeled me down the hallway and stopped by a bronze plaque that read, "Dedicated to the memory of Captain Ezekiel Hardy . . . this tablet is erected by his widow." The plaque was typical of the thousands that enshrine the memories of wealthy patrons of hospitals, churches, and so forth. The shrink asked me to read that plaque and explain it to him. I did. He concluded that this was dramatic proof that I could read. I countered that a plaque on the wall wasn't a book.

He held to his position and continued, "Fred, you can read, you just want to read better. If they cannot help you here, find a place where they can."

The idea of revolution was firmly planted in our minds. It quickly germinated to the thought of firing the entire hospital. Up the rising! Judy and I agreed that I would hang in there until she could find a better place for me to go.

The people we were running from, however, would determine where we ran to. When Cornwallis surrendered the British army at Yorktown, the American troops played a new tune, "The World Turned Upside Down." That was my situation. My world was turned upside down in my planning to leave the hospital before I was cured. I had dreams of burning my wheelchair in the parking lot the day I left. But now, in a cloud of defeat, we (the wheelchair and I) were to be consigned to another hospital. Oh well, at least I got out before Martha broke my hip.

Before the final retreat is called from my first hospital, this is an appropriate place to tell a tale or two about my nurse Martha.

Martha

Martha was the nurse who said she was "not a maid" when I asked her to make my bed go up. In retrospect, I think she may not have liked me. My first meeting with Martha had a poor beginning. Although no one would empty my urinal at night, she came in the morning as if the urinal was a magnet drawing her to it. She shook the urinal; it was empty, probably spilled at night. Then she shoved the urinal under the cover and wedged it into my crotch. She said, "Johnson, the doctor wants a urine specimen."

When I indicated that the doctor was not going to get a urine specimen, Martha sucked in her cheeks and through puckered lips hissed, "Boy, you're going to pee and if I have to throw you into the showers I will, but you will give me that urine specimen, now!" Martha did not get "her" specimen of urine or the "doctor's" specimen. Who wants to quibble over the ownership of a urine specimen anyway?

At that time, I was just out of the emergency room. My memory was poor. But the threat of throwing me into the shower cut a deep scar. What might be thought of as banal hospital chatter registered in my mind as an on-going threat.

Martha was the nurse assigned to give me showers. I had rather enjoyed showers before my stroke. Now they were a thing of terror. At any time of the day, the nurses might fall into a formation like Ral Partha harpies and descend upon us. No one could escape. We would be corralled into our rooms with the explanation that it was "time to take a shower" and be told to get fresh clothes. The nurses prodded us on with what is euphemistically called a potty chair. This chair was essentially a commode seat riveted to two pieces of aluminum tubing that sat on cheap coaster wheels. The company I had worked for was the largest producer of promotional aluminum furniture in the United

States, and I had a passing familiarity with product liability suits. Thus, I had the presence of mind to be afraid of those chairs; however, without the least bit of thought, Martha would fling me across the room in one of those chairs. Being barefoot, I think I was more afraid of stubbing my toes on the way than I was of falling.

After I was in the shower area, it was necessary to stand me up. Since the chair had no brakes, I was hesitant to stand up on a wet floor. It is generally thought that stroke patients tend to be reckless; it is not unusual to be cautioned by doctors that they may want to grab the car keys and go for a drive. I was not that reckless; my conservative attitude toward safety caused me to be terrified. One might laugh and say, "Well Fred, nothing happened; it was all in your head." It is easy enough to think that, but I still think I was fortunate to have gotten out before Martha broke my hip.

Escape

What could have been a relatively simple affair, my consignment to another hospital, quickly became a problem. It was suggested (more likely decided) that I go to Baylor University in Waco, Texas, and work in their program while receiving physical therapy at another hospital across town. We were told that the paperwork had been put in motion to effect this transfer.

On the positive side, Waco was not far from Houston, where we had family. Judy called both institutions, but each denied knowing about the arrangements. When Judy confronted the doctors with this contradictory information, she was told rather firmly that she should tend to woman's work and leave the doctor's work to the doctors. Aside from the foolish and offensive nature of the advice, the doctors' response ignored the fact that the wife of a stroke victim is going to be immediately thrust into the new role of having to take over the responsibilities her husband once carried.

The few hospitals I've been in seem to regard wives and brothers as a necessary evil. Little effort was made to take advantage of this potential pool of "free labor." Given the personnel shortages hospitals generally face, it seems reasonable to press relatives into service, especially at meal time. Yet the dining area of my first hospital had a sign posted that read, "No Visitors, Including Family."

Relatives, of course, could also make a fine addition to the proverbially overworked and understaffed transport corps within the hospital. Since a lot of effort is expended to help the stroke patient and his family re-adjust to their new circumstances, the use of family labor could further this adjustment and accomplish the aforementioned tasks.

When Judy realized that I was within an inch of being sent

to God-knows-where in Houston, she had the presence of mind to call my boss, Howard Rice, Jr. Given the similarities in their names, she was connected by mistake to Howard Rice, Sr., the president of the company I worked for. She quickly blurted out the story. Mr. Rice, a wealthy philanthropist, said, "Judy, I'll get my doctor to send over an ambulance to take Fred to Bay View [another hospital in Miami]. Hell, I give them enough money that I ought to own the place. They named a floor after me."

After a few negotiations with the social worker and a long argument with the business office about what my insurance policy would cover, I was sent to Bay View Hospital. Over the years I had skillfully side-stepped those many union demands to improve the group insurance plan, the same plan I was covered under. As the business office forcefully pointed out the deficiencies in my insurance coverage, I was to recall the biblical adage about sowing and reaping. The harvest was bitter.

Bay View

On my arrival at Bay View, there was some confusion about which room I would occupy. That problem was sorted out in short order. As I was wheeled to my room, I noticed that some of the corridors were green. I viewed this as a positive sign, since on the evening of my stroke a friend called my wife from the West Coast and asked her, "Judy, the emergency room was green, wasn't it?"

Judy replied, "I don't know, what difference does it make? Yes, it was green."

Our friend continued in her lyrical California way: "Judy, don't be afraid. Fred has been made to lie down in green pastures. The Lord will restore his soul."

Thereafter my son, Sam, read this psalm to me. With a commercial lettering set, Judy hand lettered the psalm on a piece of posterboard.

The Twenty-third Psalm seems to be exclusively reserved for graveside ceremonies at funerals. Yet it is singularly appropriate for near death situations such as strokes, and is very meaningful for me. It is reprinted below. Even if you have read it, it's worth a second perusal.

> The Lord is my shepherd; I shall not want.
> He maketh me to lie down in green pastures: he leadeth me beside the still waters.
> He restoreth my soul: he leadeth me in the paths of righteousness for his name's sake.
> Yea, though I walk through the valley of the shadow of death, I will fear no evil: for thou art with me; thy rod and thy staff they comfort me.
> Thou preparest a table before me in the presence of mine enemies: thou anointest my head with oil; my cup runneth over.

Surely goodness and mercy shall follow me all the days of
my life: and I will dwell in the house of the Lord for ever.

So I was not surprised when the room to which I was finally
assigned was plush and had a great view of Biscayne Bay. Before
I got lost in the beauty of the view, Judy and Dr. Michaels came
in.

Dr. Michaels was a slight man with brown hair who carried
about him a special radiance. In the casting of a play, he would
be a good candidate for St. Francis of Assisi. When they walked
in, I was passing a good deal of gas in a steady stream. Soon my
flatulence assumed a rat-a-tat-tat precision of an ack-ack gun at
the height of an air raid. Dr. Michaels, in his methodical way,
asked if I had had that problem before my stroke. When I indicated
that I hadn't, he asked me to stop.

I derived a great deal of pleasure from continuing. Certainly
my mother had taught me manners, yet I enjoyed breaking loose
and I had to struggle not to laugh. I was aware of the contrast
between my traditional norms of behavior and my conduct now.
I was at a loss to explain to myself the change and my lack of
will power. The disparity struck me as significant, but again I was
not sure just what it signified.

Dr. Michaels said that he wanted to run some supplemental
tests to ensure that I was in no immediate danger of a second
stroke. He courteously mentioned that some of the tests might
be repeats, because the paperwork is always mixed up in a transfer. The doctor added that the staff of the hospital would evaluate
me in order to recommend where I should go for rehabilitation
therapy.

I was immensely pleased after months of being in a quag-
mire; I had found a doctor who told me what he was going to do
up front. Not only had he told me his plan, but the plan seemed
reasonable. The business-like manner of the doctor was also reas-
suring. I abruptly returned to reality when Dr. Michaels asked me
who the president of the United States was. I was secretly amused
and proud that I knew the answer. I was amused so much that I
horsed around with the answer and said, "The actor from California." In the nick of time, Ronald Reagan's name came to mind.

Not one to leave well enough alone, the doctor asked me
who the vice-president was. I could not find the answer. Judy
chimed in and said, "Fred, you know he's from Texas!" I then
answered, "George Bush." I was pleased that Judy, who is apolit-
ical, knew who George Bush was and that he was from Texas.

Dr. Michaels continued and asked me to calculate some

numbers. "Fred, what is 86 minus 7, the remainder minus 7, and so on ad nauseam?" I started my reply with a cocky "That's no problem," but then I realized I could not answer—that part of my brain had died. As I cried out, the doctor told me not to worry about it, that I might get some of it back.

I had much to consider while the supplemental medical tests were being given to me. I now had a very pleasant place in which to consider the vast changes in my life.

In the morning, the nurses helped me dress and put me into a wheelchair to eat breakfast. The food was good. After breakfast, the nurses set me up in the hallway with an old hotel bell that would clang when struck with the palm of my hand. The bell was taped to a pillow and left in my lap. A few doors down, there was a public sitting area with a good view of Biscayne Bay. Without realizing it, I was teaching myself to use the wheelchair. As I wheeled down to the sitting area to muse over the bay and watch the gulls, I recalled that I had heard the wing beats of the Angel of Death. In the confusion and flux of my life, I thought that this escape from death might serve as a base on which to build a reasonable reaction to my stroke.

While I was in college, Viktor Frankel's book, *Man's Search for Meaning*, was quite the rage. It is the marvelous story of a Viennese psychiatrist who survived the World War II concentration camps. He wrote that when confronted with a major catastrophe, it was natural to search for a meaning. In his case, he concluded that God wanted a trained observer in the camps to tell the story. Although my account does some violence to Frankel's poetic message, it was his message that I recalled as I watched the sea gulls drift over the bay.

My life was crushed at the age of thirty-seven. Where the hell could there be meaning in that? I knew that to rebuild my life I had to have a hope, a straw to grasp at. It occurred to me that my meaning might lie in the fact that I did not die. If God had stayed the Angel of Death, it was perhaps because He had a mission, a plan, for me. Please do not marshal all of the theological counterattacks yet. If you are sitting in a hospital corridor, broken in your prime, the thought has great appeal.

If God spared me, it might be for a mission, a cause. My skills had heretofore been in the area of speaking, of talking to people. It was reasonable to believe that the mission might involve talking to people. I can talk more effectively if I can walk and have the use of my left arm. It followed, then, that it was likely in God's plan that my arm and leg would be made whole again.

For those of you with little faith, my thoughts had a certain internal consistency that was appealing. This conjecture offered me a hopeful solution. Should one object that it is presumptuous to guess God's plan? Such an objection might be a fair one, although a bit trivial. The scenario for returning to public speaking *was* a possible alternative that was attractive; hoping for it does not rule out other alternatives. Another virtue of this theory is that it reinforced my image of being "snatched back from the brink of death." This logically led to the possibility that I was reincarnated in some way. Reincarnation is not just a topic for some imaginative cocktail conversation. The philosophy served two subtle functions for me. The first is that it helped me realize that the part of my being that may have caused the stroke was dead. The second is that interpreting my stroke as a rebirth helped me accept the fact that my personality was changing and helped me bury the past.

The doctors might run tests to determine the cause of my stroke, but that was of no consequence to me since the fellow or *geist* that caused my stroke had died. A practical manifestation of this line of thought occurred months later in Texas, when a high school friend of my wife's, with whom I had almost committed a marital indiscretion before the stroke, seemed to be boycotting Judy. When I spoke to this friend on the phone, I told her there was no need to stay away, the fellow she almost had trouble with died in Florida.

Shortly before my stroke, Judy had taken a battery of self-administered psychology tests, which included the wonderful question, "Has God ever talked to you on a mountain?" Given the obvious skepticism concerning religious visions, I thought it better not to mention some of the religious insights I was having. Yet I thought the reincarnation story was a safe one, and I repeated it a few times.

I'm inclined to think that my healing process started as I watched the gulls. It was good to be in a hospital by the sea. I'm from a seaport town, and as I watched the gulls I would recall the sailor's prayer, "Oh, God, your sea is so great and my boat is so small." I often repeated the words as told in the biblical story of the flood and at the close of *Moby Dick*: "And the great shroud of the sea rolled on as it rolled five thousand years ago."

A Special Case of Worse

When Judy and Sam visited, the three of us would sneak off to the bay through the hospital's back doors and around construction sites. The hospital's expansion program was beginning to have the unhappy side effect of walling out of sight its most effective recuperative force, the bay.

The hospital's location by the bay made it difficult for Judy to visit me. The drive from our home down Interstate 95 was long and hard and crossed a congested causeway. An undercurrent of tensions began to surround her visits. Although we were not so crass as to verbalize it, we silently began to struggle with the question, "Which is worse, to have a stroke or to be married to someone who has had a stroke?"

There is little doubt in my mind as to which is the worse. I have met a few husbands whose wives had divorced them after they had a stroke. I think the almost universal reaction is, "What a cold-hearted woman!" Although my sympathies clearly lie with the stroke victim, I believe that it is all too easy to judge those wives while piously mouthing the vow, "for better or for worse." A stroke is a special case of worse and must come close to being the worst.

Judy had married an image, a dream, and a hopeful life-style when she took me on. After having done a great job of raising our only son, she now began caring for me, which was the same as getting another child when she was forty. With our son, it was always evident that he would grow up; with me, the issue was in dispute. The medical hierarchy continued to warn Judy how bleak my future was and to be prepared to just stick me in front of a television set. Judy had lost a husband and was saddled with a new child.

I felt I had betrayed my wife. When she promised the "better

33

or worse" part, I also had made a contract with her to care for her and for our unborn children. I was reneging on my part of the deal; I was betraying my family.

The ideal marriage to have before experiencing a stroke is one as strong as the "threefold cord" described by the preacher in Ecclesiastes 4: 9–12. To better understand marriage and strokes, this passage is worth a careful reading:

> Two are better than one; because they have a good reward for their labour.
> For if they fall, the one will lift up his fellow: but woe to him that is alone when he falleth; for he hath not another to help him up.
> Again, if two lie together, then they have heat: but how can one be warm alone?
> And if one prevail against him, two shall withstand him; and a threefold cord is not quickly broken.

A stroke adds a unique strain on a marriage—one that could unravel the Gordian knot, much less a threefold cord.

Although there was no specific crisis, Judy learned to fear that I might die. We can all laugh and throw our heads back and say, "Of course we are going to die." But Judy said she experienced the same unrelenting fear you carry with you after being in an auto wreck. Every time you get into a car again, you know in an immediate, deep-seated way that things can go sour.

As she was to try to build a new life with me, Judy was aware in a fundamental way that I was mortal and that our life together was at risk. I was in no obvious danger and gave the matter little thought. My reincarnation myth allowed me to believe that "the part of my being that caused the stroke is dead," therefore I was safe . . .

The Fix

Although I was not quite ready to accept a partially paralyzed leg, I knew that if I was to become a phoenix rising out of my ashes, it was time to start my rehabilitation. Dr. Michaels stated that the consultations were taking too long and that he had ordered some physical therapists to teach me some exercises to bridge the time gap.

Thus, I was not surprised one afternoon when I was taken to a therapy gym. I thought I was going to learn some exercises. But unbeknownst to me, I was being evaluated for admission to the hospital's in-house rehabilitation program. I did not realize that this hospital *had* a rehabilitation center.

I was to hear years later the cruel joke, "Do you know the prerequisite for being admitted to the XYZ therapy program?"

"Sure, money," was the answer.

That callous attitude was not being applied at Bay View (that would come later). I was not being evaluated financially, but rather to see if they thought they could help me. My understanding was that they were trying to decide where to send me, but under the guise of these exercises, I was evaluated for admission to their own program.

The entire matter was handled so obliquely that there were a few major clues I missed, though we will need to return to them eventually. I was physically evaluated by some therapists to see if I would fit into the program, but I never saw the doctor who ran the unit. He arrived at his decision based on the reports of his therapists. The matter was handled so deftly that I do not recall exactly how I learned that I was being admitted to their unit. I was working with one of the therapists at the time. With all the feigned innocence I could muster, I asked, "If they are admitting me to the unit, that means they think they can help me, doesn't it?" The reply was a smiling, "Of course."

I do not know what request my doctor had made of the hospital, but I read all sorts of meaning into the fact that I was admitted to Bay View's rehabilitation unit. As I explained to Judy with a reasoning process marred by too many years of trench warfare with unions, "Mr. Rice has given this place a lot of money. He asked them to take care of me. The safe thing to do would be to send me somewhere else. If they keep me here, they must be very sure of helping me or they run the risk of offending a wealthy patron."

For the first time since my stroke, things were looking up. Although I may have faced an uphill struggle, that was of no account, the fix was in. By accepting me at the risk of offending a donor, I thought the hospital was putting its stamp of approval on my successful recovery; it must be a sure thing. The fix was in.

I admit that I chuckle while thinking that some day a clinician will read the previous paragraph and decide to add this trait to the list of personality characteristics of stroke victims: "insecurity about the future compels them to seek assurances that everything will be all right, that the fix is in."

Rather than being a secondary characteristic of stroke victims, I feel this was merely the outgrowth of my many years in labor relations. It is fine to say, "work hard and pray," but it is a great relief if you can convince yourself that the fix is in.

As an added bonus, the therapy was being done in Miami with my family nearby. It turned out that there were no beds available in the rehabilitation area, but to me this was no problem. The transport folks could get me to the gym each day. The therapists said it was important to be in the same building with the other stroke victims. For my part, I didn't care. Stroke patients were like jails: if you've seen one, you've seen them all.

I feel the weight of the critic justifiably jumping all over my back for making such rash generalizations as, "if you've seen one, you've seen them all." I just did not understand this dormitory approach to therapy.

While I was waiting for a room, the therapists started to make a new sling for my left arm. Up to that time, I had been wearing an off-the-shelf, out-of-the-box hemi-sling for my left arm. I needed the sling not because I had broken bones, but because my bones were so heavy that they tended to pull my arm out of its socket.

The hemi-sling overcame that problem by strapping my arm across the front of my chest. This is a short-term solution to this problem and does little to retrain the sholder to hold the arm up by itself and to keep it in place. In the long run, this solution tends to freeze the bone in the socket.

The Sling

My new sling was to be a better solution. It would support my arm in the shoulder socket, thus reducing the pain, but the arm would be allowed to bounce in and out of the socket. This would keep the joint from freezing up and hopefully rekindle some interest in the shoulder muscles in reactivating themselves. My arm would pivot at the elbow, allowing for a more normal movement of the muscles and joints.

The sling began to sound like so many politicians on the stump; it promised everything. Also, like a pod of politician's promises, the sling was something to behold.

And it worked. The cradle that my left arm rested in was molded from a plastic blank. The blank was dropped into a tank of boiling water and formed to the shape of my arm. No special allowances were made for my palm, fingers, or thumb. My arm was held into the brace by Velcro strips.

The straps for the sling went over my shoulder in a rather conventional manner. It was when they connected to the plastic arm support that things got out of hand. The entire rig was hooked together by bright red elastic that looked as if it had been snipped from a balloon. The elastic allowed the arm to bounce up and down in a very limited range. This provided the needed support while keeping the shoulder joint free. With the red balloon-like elastic, however, the entire affair looked like hell.

Aside from its therapeutic effects, the dynamic sling allowed stroke patients to identify each other. When I was eventually transferred to the rehabilitation ward, the sling would act as a mark of Cain, clearly identifying those who had suffered a stroke. Although I had the habit of thinking everyone I saw in the hospital was a stroke victim, I was nevertheless hesitant to talk to strangers for fear that I would intrude upon a truly sick person. The sling tended to wear down any barriers to conversation with other stroke victims, as it marked us as part of a fellowship.

The Sergeant

My transfer to the Bay View rehabilitation unit was in the middle of the night. My meager hospital possessions were stored in a cardboard box and a paper bag. I was wheeled over to the rehabilitation center. The transport personnel got me into bed and said the head nurse would be in shortly.

Within half an hour, the night-shift head nurse, a Mrs. Sign, drifted in and introduced herself. I told her that my parents used to shoot with a colorful Army sergeant named Sign, so I should be able to remember her name. I have always been poor at names and rarely tried word association, but a head nurse was close enough to a sergeant to remember the name Sign. Nurse Sign cast a quick glance at my paper bag of clothes and asked me if it was all right for her to put them in the chest of drawers. Because I wanted to know where everything was, I asked if it was permitted for me to unpack. The nurse smiled when she realized I was willing to help. Many stroke patients would just lie back and watch, but I offered to help. Rather than being a part of a rekindled work ethic, my offer to help was rooted in a desire to start off on the right foot in the unit and to be able to find things.

When I unpacked the bag, I put a small gold-framed picture of Sam and a Gideon Bible on the dresser top. I have come to believe that nurses are more compassionate toward a patient if he is religious or a family man. I began to feel the urge to be an ideal patient, so I readily volunteered to Nurse Sign, "I know it must be difficult working with stroke patients. I'm fairly well-adjusted; if you need anyone to talk to another patient, I would be glad to help." If not broken, I had been tamed and was ready for therapy and would be submissive within tolerable limits.

In many respects, the ward looked normal except for the number of patients with dynamic slings. In the northern corner of the floor was the dining area. Cafeteria tables were clustered in the large, open room, which had a fair number of tall windows. Although not quite a sun deck, the overall effect was pleasing. The room did not seem to be a part of the ward. There were no lively posters proclaiming "There is no gain without pain!" Although I've heard it often, I do not believe this old saw of football is true for hospital wards.

I had thought that stroke patients were clustered together in this ward to accomplish some cheap psychological sleight of hand. I resented that someone thought I would take solace in the fact that there were people who had it worse than me. I would have done well to recall Father Hugh Kennedy's wisdom in Edwin O'Connor's *The Edge of Sadness* (New York: Little, Brown & Company, 1962, p. 207):

> "I mean when you cut your hand off, it hurts; it doesn't hurt any less simply because a thousand other people may have cut their hand off before you."
> "No, but if you remember all those other hands you may be prevented from hiring a hall and giving a short talk on 'How I cut my hand off.' It helps you keep a sense of proportion. Otherwise, you begin to fondle your own personal catastrophes and that seems dangerous to me."

Although I did gain a good deal of perspective from the dorm effect, I suspect the writing of this book may be viewed as the equivalent of hiring a hall and giving a short talk on how I had a stroke.

We were encouraged to eat together in the day room. One tangible result of this was that there would always be someone's relative present to help unbundle my food. I never mastered the art of opening a milk carton with one hand. The plastic silverware could be removed from its cellophane pack by holding it loosely in your fist and striking the table with it. By using my knife as a wedge, I could get the flip-top tab of a soft drink can started up and finish the job with my right hand.

After breakfast, I wheeled back to my room to wait for transport to take me to therapy. Physical therapy was on the first floor. With my diminished sense of direction, I thought it was in the basement since it was at the bottom of the elevator shaft; I forgot that there are few basements in Miami Beach. Although called a gym, there was little in the therapy room that suggested a typical gym. There were a number of low tables covered with red mats. The therapists seemed to be wrestling with the patients on these mats. Rather than having an audience on the bleachers, this gym's spectators were a row of elderly patients in wheelchairs next to a set of parallel bars.

My physical therapist found me and wheeled me to a mat. I looked wistfully at the parallel bars, silently suggesting, "Let's practice walking." With no words of explanation, the therapist firmly replied, "Fred, you cannot walk." I emphatically denied this, pleading, "I walked at the other hospital." Her reply was a curt, "We may be able to help you, but you cannot walk."

My level of frustration increased on the merry-go-round of "if you can walk." As I have come to understand it, this dispute did not really involve my physical abilities, but instead was centered in the philosophy of my treatment. The reader may tire of my "as I have come to understand it," and request that I do my homework and give a definitive answer. Let's be fair. To paraphrase a statement made in the Watergate hearings: I'm telling you what I knew and when I knew it.

There are two contrasting theories of physical therapy for stroke victims, although both agree that therapy should begin as soon as possible after the stroke. (There may be other theories, but these are the two I know about.) The first school of thought might be characterized with the statement, "Stand them up, slap a brace on them, and get them walking." The other school, which was followed at Bay View, stressed the gradual building up of muscle groups and thought that any premature effort at walking would set back the entire program. A follower of the second school would say that my walking was under such poor control that it was doomed to fail. Thus, I could not walk in any real sense. This is not some esoteric scholarly argument; it was woven into the fabric of my treatment program.

One might ask, "Fred, having experienced both schools of treatment, which do you feel is better?" I would be inclined to duck the question, for I do not know a positive answer. If you feel compelled to protest that I would not be able to make a simple either/or choice, imagine my feelings of uncertainty during the treatment. For me, it was not six of one or a half-dozen of the other. I wanted a definite answer to the gray question of which was better, yet there is no proven answer.

For me, the issue was not framed by the consideration that one type of therapy must be better than the other. The basic question was the haunting, "Will I walk?" The realization that there were two different schools of thought on this prompted the nagging speculation that maybe I would walk better or sooner, or more certainly, if I got the other type of therapy!

There was no way to ignore the "two schools" issue. At

coffee break, the therapists would make mention of their personal preference for a certain technique of the opposing school. They would generally say, "If it works, I will use it," in a hushed tone, as if they were embarrassed at saying a good word about the other method of treatment. It was akin to a chiropractor admitting that aspirin may kill pain. That the therapists were discussing my treatment and how to better it might have evoked a positive reaction from me; rather, it served to remind me that there was another, and perhaps more efficacious, method of treatment.

Since walking was ruled out, the exercises in physical therapy were rather imaginative, the goal being to work specific muscle groups. Bear in mind that paralysis is caused because the brain is not sending impulses to the nerves to activate the muscles. I began to believe in acupuncture when the therapist would touch a trigger point on my arm with a vibrator, and my hand would move. Equally impressive was the fact that she told me it would move before it did.

My arm could work if I could get my brain in gear. As I cried in attempts to move the unmovable, I recalled the endless taunts that Sister Mary Genuflex used to make about the million brain cells I was wasting. Those verbal floggings usually came when I failed a spelling test. I failed enough spelling tests that I should have had all those millions of brain cells held ready in reserve, but I could not turn them on. It is not as if the stroke had killed them all, the remainder just were not plugged in.

In my frustration about my arm, I fabricated my own Faustian myth (replacing the devil with God), and as if driven like Coleridge's Ancient Mariner, I would tell my therapist, "I don't know why I'm telling you this story; it isn't true, but I feel compelled to tell you. I made a deal with God that if He gives me my left leg back, I will forgo my left arm."

Now, of course, that never really happened, for surely I could negotiate a better deal than that of an arm for a leg. To repeat, I never struck such a bargain with God or with the devil. Why I felt compelled to tell people that I had made such a deal is not yet clear to me. When I would despair about my left arm, my occupational therapist would quietly and cunningly ask me if I wanted to give up on the left arm. In spite of any deal, real or imagined, I always replied that I wanted to continue therapy on my left arm.

"Occupational therapy" was one of the seemingly self-explanatory terms that I ran across in the rehabilitation process that could be misleading. The thrust of the occupational therapy department was to help the patient be self-sufficient at home. In my case, I think my work in the department went well because I only vaguely grasped its goals and approached it as a boondoggle.

The occupational therapy department was next to physical therapy, but the two departments were connected by a door. There was a mat in one corner of the occupational therapy room with a well-stocked kitchen in another. Since I received physical therapy in the occupational therapy area, the idea came to mind that the separation of the two areas just might have something to do with a double insurance payment, since the two departments were separately staffed.

Before I could begin to feel sorry for the insurance companies, my wife asked me to sign a boilerplate agreement that we would be liable, and pay, for my speech rehabilitation if my insurance company did not. In response to the immediate question of why the insurance company would not pay for my speech rehabilitation, my speech pathologist, Annalisa Archer, replied that insurance companies were hesitant to pay for services that were not performed by a doctor. With her master's degree and years of experience, Annalisa certainly was qualified. She had even written a basic sourcebook for the treatment of aphasics. There followed a round of my obligatory observations that anyone who could pronounce "Annalisa Archer" did not need a speech pathologist. And why *was* I having a speech pathologist instead of a therapist?

The next round of my insurance problem introduced me to the unit social worker, Bruce Mendez. I was white and middle class; for me, the title "social worker" carried with it a lot of negative connotations. Bruce told Judy that I was to be discharged in six days because my insurance was running out. Since I was the patient desperate for treatment and had a mind destabilized by the stroke, the hospital business office was disinclined to believe me when I told them that my insurance was not about to run out. In spite of all the moans and groans the unions had raised about the insurance policy, I knew it was not *that* shabby. I just had to find a spokesperson the hospital would believe. Judy called an executive I knew in the administrative offices of the insurance company. He wrote a rather unusual letter to the hospital on insurance company letterhead that unequivocally stated that the insurance company would pick up the tab.

The Dorm Effect

The social worker lurked in the background to act as a catalyst for the "dorm effect." In the foreground, no doctor was in sight. Vincent Garabaldi, the doctor who ran the rehabilitation unit, seemed to be an absentee boss.

Mornings were rushed. Breakfast trays were brought to the room to be picked at while dressing. Aside from the expected problems, dressing was slowed down by having to put on a pair of special shoes. Everyone in the unit wore high-top tennis shoes, with the front part split open so that a hard rubber bridge could be placed under the toes and heels.

The irony of having special shoes when it was anathema to walk was not lost on me. But not until I left the hospital did I dare ask about this seeming contradiction. I was given the rather reasonable explanation that although we did not walk in our type of therapy, we spent a good deal of time on our feet. The reason our heels and toes were elevated was to create an extended muscle pattern in the leg when and if we put weight on our feet.

Hopefully when breakfast was done, someone from transport would arrive to wheel me to physical therapy. At the nurses' station by the elevator we would pick up my chart. My chart was a rather large loose-leaf notebook. On the ride down, I would page through my chart, though most of the notes were not legible. In the upper right-hand corner of one report, a black-and-white Polaroid photograph was taped. It was the type of photograph taken of the viewing screen of an imaging machine. I jumped to the conclusion that the picture was a cross-section image of my brain. It looked like a slice of watermelon with seeds scattered throughout. I concluded that the seeds represented parts of my brain that were dead. My visualization of my brain as the photo of a slice of watermelon simplified that brain to a one-dimensional slab, all pock-marked with dead sections.

I soon learned that the physical therapists did not approve of patients reading their charts.

The folks in occupational therapy were more relaxed about such things. Their less up-tight, casual manner of business might once have dismayed me, but my obsession for order was relaxing and I needed a break after the stringent physical therapy. In occupational therapy I had no burning obsession, such as walking, to drive me on. It was just a pleasant place to go after physical therapy and do another set of exercises.

But once again, as if realizing one of the fantasies of my teenage years, I was hovered over by a band of beautiful—amazingly beautiful—women. And, of course, it was fate that one of the warmer, more beautiful, and more personable of these women, Beckie Brown, was to be my therapist. All the aspects of my therapy were coordinated to accomplish my rehabilitation and all had their value. The whole, indeed, is not greater than the sum of its parts. Thus it is perhaps not fair to single out occupational therapy or Beckie, for she was not the only therapist I was to have a crush on. Later, I will speak of Jane, April, and Lynne. So many have helped, and the road was long. But I *will* single out Beckie.

My introduction to Beckie lost some of its glitter when we were ten minutes into our first exercise and I told her I had to urinate. This was no easy task. The bathroom in the therapy area was on a narrow corridor that served as the collective storage area for physical and occupational therapy. In the hall were all the file cabinets and junked desks of the two departments.

It seemed an intentional obstacle course, with the relief of one's bladder as the prize for successfully navigating it. Getting to the door of the bathroom was not enough, for the resistance setting of the automatic door return was set on high. The junk in front of the door necessitated rolling to the door sideways, and it was nearly impossible to kick the door open. On this day, as the door swung shut, my left arm could not fend it off, and my chair was firmly wedged between the closing door and the door casement.

I was desperate, but I was not about to wet my pants in front of Beckie on the first day I had met her. At the appropriate moment, though, she intervened and helped with the door. By the time I was finished, it was time to go to speech pathology. With a balanced delicacy, Beckie held my hand and placed her other under my chin to turn my face to her. She looked gently into my eyes and said, "Fred, we lost all of our exercise time going to the bathroom. Next time please try to take care of those things before you come down." My emotions were so frayed that a less gentle rebuke would have been devastating.

Although Beckie seemed disappointed about it, the cutting short of my exercise time did not seem of great consequence to me. I did not think that I would need to have a certain number of hours of a particular set of exercises under my belt to be able to walk. I thought more in terms of being in the rehabilitation unit for an extended period of time. If one particular exercise was rained out, there was always tomorrow. Rather than labeling my attitude as lackadaisical, it is more accurate to say that I was lazy. Thus, I was happy to learn that Beckie considered our wheeling around the corridors an exercise to help me regain my sense of direction and space perception. Rather than thinking of this as therapy, I, of course, considered it to be a magnificent waste of time that allowed me to speak with this charming young woman.

On one of our walks, with deeper perception than I realized I had at the time, I asked Beckie and myself, "When do I cease to be a stroke victim?" My answer, sadly enough, was that I would be a stroke victim until the day "my Lord and Savior may make me whole as He sees fit." The quality of my life was improving at Bay View, yet I was not whole, and until then I was a victim. It looked as if I would be a victim for a long time. With a disarming grace, Beckie would duck my question, "How long?" In a mere act of raising the issue, I had started to think the unthinkable. Although I was not willing to accept a compromise and throw in the towel, I was sensing the answer to "how long" might be a very long time.

Although I regarded our working together in the hallways as a pleasant diversion, it *did* seem as if our practice was yielding results. If it had not been too complex, I could retrace the steps of the prior day's journey with little prompting. The corridors of the various hospital buildings were all color coded. Rather than leaning forward to follow a painted stripe on the floor, I just had to be alert to the color of the walls. If the color changed, I knew I was at an intersection of corridors and had to find a sign for guidance. That being done, I could follow the arrow to thread my way through the intersection. Although I was getting better, I navigated on one horizontal plane only—the ground floor.

Elevators were an obstacle because of my fear that the small front wheel of the chair would lodge in the crack of the shaft. Wheelchairs generally fold up so they can be placed in car trunks. The accordion effect that might result from being caught in a wheelchair between renegade elevator doors struck me as a real threat. Beckie was perceptive enough not to ask me if I was afraid of elevators. One morning she told me that we were going to work on elevators, and as it was so often with occupational therapy, this was a pleasant, unexpected diversion.

The trick turned out to be to go into the elevator straight on. If the chair is facing the elevator door, the front wheels of the chair cannot be angled and get lodged in or fall into the crack of the shaft. Once safely in, I concentrated on the buttons to the side of the doors, ignoring the lights above the doors that indicated the true position of the elevator. Unmindful that people above and below could influence where the elevator went, I acted as if the machine were my slave. If the door opened, I wheeled out in a rush to avoid the doors. My getting off on the right floor was a happy coincidence. When I got off on the wrong floor, I soon realized it, and the panic of geographic disorientation would overwhelm me.

As Beckie helped me understand the nature of my mistake, I began to watch the row of lights above the doors. The entire matter would have been simplified if the hospital had stenciled floor numbers in large digits on the walls facing the elevator doors. It looks tacky, but it would have helped.

As my elevator skills improved, Beckie carefully reviewed with me the route from my room to the physical therapy gym. At first, there seemed little reason for this exercise. After all, the transport staff took me wherever I needed to go.

Although there may be similarities and common characteristics among stroke victims, each of us is unique. Many of the other patients on the floor did not have my acute geographic disorientation or fear of falling down the elevator shaft. These more agile patients did not have to wait for personnel from transport to take them to therapy in the morning or to return them in the afternoon. The transport staff, however, was exquisitely slow, and I often waited a long time for their help. The more agile patients avoided this and were able to return to their rooms and take a nap.

After realizing all the advantages of getting around by oneself, I decided one morning to try to to go to therapy by myself. My journey was successful and uneventful. This was a significant step in my rehabilitation. I functioned on my own and curbed my quick and facile excuse, "Oh, I don't want to learn to be institutionalized. Teach me to *walk* to therapy."

My going to therapy independently had been an unannounced goal; Beckie had not given it to me to work toward. It was a happy and predictable by-product of our therapy. Avoiding the wait for transport was sufficient incentive. Being able to take a nap was a reasonable reward for a quick return from therapy.

I had come a long way. Just months before, at the first hospital, I would get lost in the hallway on the journey back to my room from therapy. Upon my eventual, frustrated arrival, I would be tied into my wheelchair. I received little help and scant motivation to learn to help myself. I felt proud of my new-found ability to get somewhere on my own in the wheelchair, proud but not cocky.

When I learned that Joan Felt, a secretary at the company where I worked, was in Bay View, I asked Beckie to come with me during the day to find Joan's room so I could retrace my steps at night to visit her. Joan was in the main building of the hospital. This had been my goal many times in my work with Beckie, and I expected no trouble in finding Joan's room.

The practice run was useful, although I had no problem getting to the building. The floor plan was erratic and without prior tutoring, I would have had trouble finding the room. Thus, I was reasonably confident when I set out one evening to visit Joan before supper. Although I was cutting it close on time, I thought things were well in hand. To be on the safe side, however, I told the staff at the nurses' station where I was going.

Joan was in the hospital to receive chemotherapy for cancer. I was not confident that she would be receptive to my normal pep talk that it could be worse, we could be dead. But I thought I'd try to cheer her up.

Joan was on a "high-class" floor where coffee and tea were served at three-thirty in the afternoon. We visited and shared coffee hour together. Joan was delighted at my joy when I discovered that the coffee was real, with caffeine.

I had not budgeted my time well and even though I made a quick return to my ward, a cooling dinner tray was already on my bedside table. An unfriendly nurse I did not recognize descended on me from the nurses' station. I expected a mild dressing down about being late for supper, but instead I received a major dressing down for leaving the floor without signed permission from my doctor. My first defense was that I left the floor every morning to go to therapy. The nurse was not swayed and continued her tongue-lashing by asking the standard question, "What if something happened to you?" As I remained undaunted, the nurse broached the real issue and asked, "What if Dr. Michaels or Dr. Garabaldi had come looking for you, and we did not know where you were?"

I responded, "If Dr. Michaels had been looking for me, I would have seen him in Joan's room; she is his patient. I would have been sorry to miss Dr. Garabaldi, but I doubt that he would be looking for me, he keeps such a low profile."

The nurse wandered away still grumbling that I had best get my doctor's written permission to leave the floor.

I was able to cope with this rebuke by mentally removing myself from the situation and wondering who this strange nurse could be. She must be on rotation and not know how the unit operates. Or maybe she had been exposed to too many hospital regulations to think that I needed permission from my doctor to leave the floor, as if I were sick. The nurse's lecture also ran against the current of the therapy. For months I had been withdrawn and feeling sorry for myself. When I finally vitalized some of the skills that would help me cope, my reward was a cold supper and a heated lecture.

Of course, prior to my stroke I would have shrugged my shoulders at the notion that rolling around in a wheelchair was a skill. Perhaps being more charitable now, I can recognize that it is fair to regard such commonplace things as getting around in a wheelchair or operating an elevator to be "skills." No matter how restricted or less charitable my definition of skill had been, I was now going to have to also work on the most rudimentary skills in the areas of reading, writing, and arithmetic. I had realized all along that I had a problem with reading. While in speech pathology, however, I learned that I also had deficits in math and in writing.

"Deficits" is a jarring word, like "skill." Deficits had been the sorry state of the federal budget brought on by free-spending Democrats; for me, deficits, rather than being fiscal, were now physical and mental. For me they represented things I once did, but no longer could do.

Speech pathology was a part of the rehabilitation program at Bay View. Usually a speech pathologist is associated with aphasia, the loss of the ability to speak. My paralysis is on the left side of my body, which means that the right side of my brain was damaged in the stroke. Although I thought I stuttered when I spoke, I felt sure that I was not aphasic, which is usually a problem when the stroke occurs on the left side of the brain. I was not, however, seeing the speech pathologist, Annalisa Archer, because of my stutter, real or imagined. From Annalisa (who, like all speech pathologists, was a beautiful woman) I learned that I had many problems associated with aphasia.

In the beginning, my speech rehabilitation was limited to enunciating Kaputaka and Nantucket. When we moved on to writing, I promptly related my anecdote about not being able to spell and that my handwriting was indecipherable. To encourage me to try to write, we agreed that I would write letters to my parents. Each day Annalisa would review the letter I had written the day before and have me search for errors she caught and have me correct them. But even after I made the corrections, my letters still lacked a good deal of content. There was also no notation to warn my parents that these were sanitized letters. This would have been appropriate since my parents might compare the letters to those written by my sister following her stroke.

Yes, my sister had a stroke. There is no need to turn back to chapter one, my bane is: a) a family history of strokes, b) high blood pressure, c) a smoking habit, and d) a stressful job. I'm nothing short of a walking advertisement for the American Heart Association.

Aside from the letters to my parents, I daily wrote a page in a green spiral notebook. (The paper was easier to control in this type of notebook.) I have had countless doctors tell me to work with my left arm so that I could use it to anchor a regular, single piece of paper while writing. I had another goal in mind. One night, when Judy was eating supper with me at the first hospital, a scruffy-looking man with whom we were sharing the table looked down at his paralyzed arm and sighed, "The first day that it works, I'm going to reach down and grab me a handful of balls."

Yes, it would have been nice if my left arm could have held down paper. In the interim, I used the spiral notebook. I still have that notebook; it is at the back of the top drawer of my red filing cabinet. I felt no compelling reason to keep the thing, and I certainly did not save it to mark how far I have come. I remember *that* all too well. Having survived one move from Florida to Texas, the notebook is more like a college term paper, hardly worth having, but on hand too long to throw away.

One afternoon Annalisa asked me if I could write the numerical equivalent of a group of multi-digit numbers. I immediately chimed in, "Yes." I was delighted at this seemingly easy homework. The list had a dozen multi-digit numbers, some of them written out, such as "one million and nine hundred." Other numbers were in arabic numerals, such as "350910" and "74321042." My task was the apparently simple one of going from words to numerals and from numerals to words. I tried, but I could not do it. I had no feel for tens or hundreds in digits; the decimal part of me was gone. This is a serious loss, but I did not experience the depression that I had felt when I found that I could not read. My ambivalent attitude was due to what I regarded as the whimsical nature of the problem. I might have lost my decimal sense, or the trouble could have been a visual one involving my inability to see the patterns of numbers or the groupings of zeros.

The entire matter was not clear to me. With more confidence than I felt, I would smile and say, "My company is tough; I don't need to understand big numbers at negotiations, one digit is enough!" My reaction was not entirely a false bravado; rather than being terrified, I was curious as to what could cause the problem. I still had my sense of magnitudes and knew that a thousand was ten times one hundred. I had a partial mastery of such things and was fascinated by my inability to comprehend multi-digit numbers in numeric form.

Roommates

When I transferred into the rehabilitation unit, I had no roommate and enjoyed a virtually private room. It is considered ill-advised to let stroke patients have private rooms. Thus, even though there were vacant rooms on the floor, I was certain to be assigned a roommate from among the new arrivals. I usually hesitated at my door each time I returned in order to listen for any signs of a roommate. To ensure that I had stopped at the right door, I had taped to the door a Kermit the Frog postcard my sister had sent me. It was easier to remember Kermit than to recall the room number.

When my new roommate finally arrived, he was with complete entourage. Transport personnel were depositing my new roommate, Sol Gold, plus full baggage. Sol was a frail man of about sixty, and he was accompanied by his wife, Karen.

I immediately launched into one of my "good patient" speeches to indirectly court Mrs. Gold by telling Sol, "It's not bad here; the food is good but you have to work or they exile you to a nursing home." With more anger in his hand than in his words, Sol cursed and shook his fist at me. I was at a loss to understand why my charm had failed. Mrs. Gold appeared so nice and petite that I had a difficult time envisioning him, with such a personality, as her husband.

As I had undergone personality changes, so had Sol, but more so. He had his stroke while under a surgeon's knife during a heart by-pass operation; he came out mad at the world. Sol's attitude was to be expected since he was aphasic.

Aphasic and aphasia both mean the loss or impairment of language. "Aphasia" is a noun; "aphasic" can be an adjective or a noun. The two words eternally juxtapose themselves. It is not as if you had an ulcer; aphasia is not something you have, it is what you are—a totality. Sol was aphasic and lost his command of language. Sol could read and follow conversation, but he could not speak, although he could curse with some fluency. This was one of the perplexing paradoxes of Sol's problem. He could not speak, but he could curse. His cursing, or automatic speech, was not a sign that he could talk.

In a dissimilar vein, I had some automatic responses that also seemed paradoxical. If I would yawn, my arm would move up so I could cover my mouth and my hand would turn out flat to cover my lips. In spite of this movement, my arm was paralyzed. In spite of his cursing, Sol could not speak.

TV Wars

Although he had lost his mastery over language, Sol enjoyed television. Our color set was mounted on the wall, and it was activated by a control built into the bed railing. To turn it off, all channels had to be rotated to the end, then the set would die at the last channel. Holding the channel selector down too long would allow you to jump past the off position to the next endless cycle of channels.

Sol and I were locked into a continual disagreement about when the set should be off. Neither of us had a burning passion about the shows to watch when the set was on, yet it seemed to me that he wanted the set on all the time. In spite of my magic watch, I still had some time disorientation and often thought the hour was much later than it actually was. Rather than asking Sol if I could turn the set off because I thought it was late, I would run through the channels to get to the dead-end channel to turn the set off.

At the start of the process, I imagine Sol did not know if I was trying to change the channel or to turn the set off. When it became obvious that I was trying to turn the set off, he would curse, press the channel selector, and the spiral would continue. If Sol's anger was fine-tuned, rather than cursing, he would throw his urinal at me. The TV was not on too late, I was just not aware of the time even though I had a digital clock on my nightstand.

One day while I was at therapy, the "electrical inspector" for the hospital unplugged my clock and "red-tagged" the cord. It was against hospital policy for patients to plug in a "private electrical appliance." My clock was a prohibited "private electrical appliance."

When our arguments became loud enough, a nurse would intervene. I expected the hospital to have a policy to resolve such disputes; however, all our nurse would tell me was that she could not turn off the TV and that I would have to work it out with Sol.

Thomas Jefferson believed that if reasonable people sat down together they could resolve any conflict by discussion. Sol and I could not sit down and reason together since he could not speak. It seems silly that a hotshot labor negotiator could not strike a bargain with this man over when to watch TV.

A Good Patient

My problems with Sol weighed heavily on my spirit; I did not want to detract from my self-image as a good patient, an image I had worked hard to build with the hospital crew. I was well-adjusted and coping well. Whether or not it was a deception, the image had to be maintained.

When you are asked, "How are you?" one suspects the questioner is soliciting a positive answer. The reply should be, "Doing well," not a long and boring listing of your troubles. On occasion, the words "all things considered" can be added to a weak "I'm doing well." Although I was not coping too well with Sol's outbursts, I thought it best not to mention that fact to anyone.

Jealousy

Since I was not aphasic, the speech and language rehabilitation program I received was different from the program laid out for Sol. Since we both had a bum arm and leg, his physical therapy was much the same as mine. In spite of the prohibition against walking, I saw Sol working on the parallel bars one day. He did well.

I was fiercely jealous of Sol's success. Sol was caught in the unimaginable grief of aphasia, yet I begrudged him his triumph on the bars.

When I had the stroke, I did not recall asking, "Why me, why not the lady down the block who is committing adultery?" I had avoided the "why not them" stage, but now I jumped to the "why not me" syndrome. I worked hard and made every effort and wanted a sign. Perhaps there was only so much of this magic healing dust to go around. Why not me instead of this grumpy old man? I realized that my jealousy was most likely a natural reaction. Still, I was ashamed and thought there must be a secret closet to hide it in. I did not hide it too well, for soon Sol and I were again locked into an open conflict over the TV. This time when he threw his urinal at me, it was not empty. Most of the time, I despaired and talked to Judy. She suggested I ask for a new roommate. Since I thought this would tarnish my image, I resisted. When my resistance was finally dampened, I asked the nurse how I could transfer to a different room. She wrote up a note and said it would take a while.

It was done. Knowing the change was in store was the balm that made it easier for me to bear up. I did not have the courtesy to tell Mrs. Gold of my treachery. In a few weeks I had a new roommate, Nathan Fine. If Sol's name was mentioned to me, I would say we were divorced.

Hamburgers

One day while eating a hamburger for lunch, I was struck by the fact that they were being served to us in white Styrofoam packages similar to the ones served at the drive-in windows of fast-food restaurants. Many of the other patients were having hamburgers that day, and I had the thought that the lunch had been catered by Burger King. Coveting another burger, and with the hope that the order had been messed up, I wheeled to the dietitian's office.

Next to the door was a rack of trays holding several hamburgers. My spirits lightened. Not only was I able to get another hamburger that day to satisfy my immediate need, but I also learned that if I wrote my request on the daily menu selection form, I could get a hamburger almost any time—just as long as I included with it a green vegetable.

Although the food was good, I embraced the chance to avoid a fricassee of this or cubes of that. I could have *real* food, such as hamburgers. For this reward I had to work. The hamburgers were not provided automatically; I had to request them from the menu. Not being sure if this was a privilege or a right, I would write on the menu, "A hamburger, please, thank you."

In this subtle way, I was learning again to influence my fate. Certainly there was a hedonistic side to the hamburger matter, but there was a planned purpose, just as encouraging my wheeling back to my room alone was a bit more than avoiding the wait for transport. I was being encouraged "to cope" in a safe and supportive environment. When I wrote "hamburger, please," I was not learning to cook a meal for myself, but I was learning to influence the future. I had a certain degree of control and was less the cripple for it.

Showers

Showers had been a time of terror at the first hospital. At Bay View they were pleasant, but attainable only after the most delicate of negotiations. There was a sign-up sheet for showers on a clipboard at the nurses' station. I always signed up for evening showers and continued to receive the "wait for the morning" dodge. In frustration, I asked the evening-shift nurse if she would give me a shower. She said she had promised to do a lady at eight o'clock and would give me one at nine. When the night-shift nurses were not busy, they would give patients showers, but you had to ask, not just sign up.

The routine that evolved for getting an evening shower would start in the morning with asking the linen clerk for an extra towel and a bar of soap. These had to be hidden during the day (of course, the hiding place would have to be remembered later), so that the hospital staff did not take them away during their daily routine.

After supper, a nurse would be asked to assist with the showers. I felt it wise to spread the burden around; thus, I had to remember who I had asked the prior evening. Between that and remembering to sign up and remembering where the towels and soap were hidden, a fair amount of mental sequencing was done just to get to the shower door. No doubt it could be said that I was showing initiative and learning to cope. It seemed, however, like I was the puppet and the hospital machine was the master, and it was not for me to see its strings. The roadblocks to getting the shower may have been a therapeutic effect, but I cannot conclude for sure that they were part of a well-planned, subtle scheme to help me. Maybe it was all happenstance.

Learning the mechanics of how to take a shower had direct benefits as part of the coping process. The shower was in a central area behind the elevator shafts. After gathering my secreted towel and soap and a clean set of pajamas, I would take my shoes off and head for the shower room, avoiding the nurses' station. Nurses have a strong aversion to patients in their bare feet. Hopefully, the nurse I had a rendezvous with would be there.

The shower room contained two showers. One was for the truly immobile; it was a galvanized tub with overhead rails on which ran a hoist and tackle.

There was a bench at the rear of the room where the more agile might sit and strip before a shower. This bench was invariably cluttered with the damp and bunched-up towels the prior user had left behind. Since a nurse was almost always present when the showers were in use, the soiled leavings of the last nurse supervising showers brought caustic comments from the nurse currently in the showers.

I would park my wheelchair by the bench, lock my wheels, check that they were locked, stand up by using the right arm of my chair for support, and then drop my shorts and underwear. Then I would get back into the chair and wheel to the shower.

The shower was like a tub with high sides that had been tiled. A grab bar was mounted vertically on the front wall of the shower. A shower seat was in the middle of the tub, and the seat had a foam-padded back which formed a chair-like structure.

After parking by the shower chair, I would go through the previously mentioned ritual of locking my wheels and double checking them. I would then grasp the bar and come to a half standing position. The nurse would pull out the right arm of my wheelchair and slap me on the butt to pivot me to the right so I would be over the edge of the shower chair. I would lower myself to its edge, and the nurse would pull back my wheelchair.

I was left with my two legs over the side of the tub. I slid onto the chair and got my legs into the tub by crossing them at the ankles and using my good right leg to drag up the left leg. A physical therapist might object to lifting the bad leg with the good one; the night-shift nurse yielded to the more practical demands of the moment.

There was no wall-mounted shower head; bathing was done with a hand-held applicator. The nurse would spray, and I would try to get the hospital soap to lather with my one good hand. Toward the end, I would rinse myself off. Drying the tub was more important than drying me. I needed a safe surface to stand on. Initially, I would want to grasp the grab bar to stand up, unmindful that I could not step out of the tub. Experience taught me, though, to swing my legs out first. Then I could stand up. The nurse would scoot the chair under me, and I would put on my pajamas, give some sincere thanks, go back to my room, put on some shoes, and go exploring down the hall.

Rights and Lefts

In occupational therapy I did not work exclusively with Beckie, but occasionally with a young woman named Karen who had polio and was fitted with metal braces. She walked with Canadian canes; Canadian canes have a metal clasp-like attachment to support the forearm and a post to hold on to.

Being cynical, I thought that Karen was in the unit as a potential role mode. Aside from being an excellent role model, she was a good therapist. At first, our therapy seemed limited to children's games. Karen would line up wooden blocks that had a diamond cut into the tops of them and ask me to duplicate the pattern. For a few days we just built little block walls and then Karen demurely said, "Fred, I think you have mirror vision."

Karen laid out a small pattern of blocks in an effort to show me I was having trouble with my perception of left and right. Mirror vision is not some diabolic super power with which I was blessed; it was another nuisance with which I was cursed. My ability to tell left from right was impaired.

I still realized which was my own right hand, but when someone was in front of me I was hard pressed to identify his or her right or left hand. This inability to reverse the images (thus the mirror label) struck me as trivial at first, and I flippantly observed that knowing people's lefts from rights was only important for separating the married women from the unmarried ones in bars.

To keep my false bravado in check, Karen told me that mirror vision would impede me in many ways. I could not follow the threading of nuts and bolts or comprehend counterclockwise, nor would I be able to work with machines.

I was never much of a mechanic and was undaunted. I was secretly pleased when Karen mentioned mirror vision. I welcomed a label. If it has a label, perhaps it could be fixed. Any type of vision problem might account for my reading difficulties and make them more socially acceptable.

The therapy I received to help my visual perception involved working with games that had patterns. I was jarred to see that the boxes were labeled for children four to six months old.

Aside from my mirror vision, I was having other perceptual problems. I tended to ignore or not be aware of things to my bad (left) side. I do not think my impairment was that severe. The classical example of this problem is of a man who only eats what is on the right side of his plate because he does not "see" the peas on the left side. He will eat them if the plate is rotated. Since I don't recall any nurses rotating my half-picked-over plate, I have to assume my neglect was not that severe. If I am not aware of the world to the left, I am not aware that I am unaware of it, but aware of it or not, there is a world that will make itself known even if I tend to ignore it. The pain of too many banged knees in doorways from misguided wheelchairs forcibly reminded me that there was a world to the left even if I ignored it. My continual running into door jambs was explained as being caused by a loss of my peripheral vision. There was talk of "field cuts." I was unable to see some areas in front of me, and the peripheral vision could be compensated for if I rotated my head using my good right eye to do the seeing. I made that adjustment naturally.

As I compensated for my visual field cuts and loss of peripheral vision by rotating my head, it soon became clear that my neglect involved many things outside the realm of optics and sight. See it or not, I tended to ignore the left side of my body. When shaving I would leave patches of whiskers on my left chin. When dressing, my left collar was never quite squared away. When I dress, I never seem to get my pants high enough up on my left side to please Judy.

When writing, I would not maintain my left-hand margins. Not maintaining left-hand margins is the expression I continually use and the one speech pathologists use. Yet when examining my writing samples post-stroke, I think it is more accurate to say that I drifted off to the right.

It is not unusual to see signs above a stroke patient's bed on his good side that read, "Speak to the patient on this side." Although the stroke patient could lose his hearing during a stroke, those signs are to guard against problems with a patient's neglect of one side. Even though the patient is not deaf, he may not notice you if you approach him from his bad side.

One of the more bizarre aspects of this type of neglect was

described by Dr. Oliver Sacks in his thoroughly enjoyable *The Man Who Mistook His Wife for a Hat*. His clinical tale about the man who fell out of bed relates the story of a man who was not aware his leg was his own. Fortunately, I did not have the bizarre problem of not knowing my own body parts. Oddly enough, however, six years after my stroke, I began to notice a phantom sensation of movement in my bad arm. I had been working with the arm steadily over the years and it was showing improvement, but not enough to independently move. The sensation of motion was so real that it was with the greatest restraint that I did not jerk my head to see the long-awaited miracle.

A stroke is a cruel, wholly un-Godly thing. There is nothing in it that is humorous. However at times, Judy and Sam will marvel and laugh at how I do things to compensate for my left-side neglect. Under no circumstances will I reach my good arm across my bad side. If I am sitting in a chair with a phone off to my left and the phone rings, rather than reach across my bad side with my good right arm, I will stand up, pivot to the right, and answer the phone.

My Amigo (a motorized cart) has a swivel seat. When I am getting out of it, I will always swivel to the right.

When considering the bizarre manifestations of neglect, it is easy to lose sight of the courage of stroke victims. When standing at a curb, you handle steps up and down by following a formula that would delight the most puritanical preacher. The formula for doing steps is the secret of getting to heaven: It is down with the bad, up with the good. You go up a step with your good foot and down with the bad one. When at a curb, you step down with your bad foot. Yet, given the perceptual problems described above, it is fair to describe this simple motion of stepping down as equivalent to Columbus's ship sailing continually on the edge of the unknown. Certainly there are monsters and great peril down there.

The Vestibular
Nervous System

I would become very frustrated while doing perception exercises and welcomed the break when Karen asked me if I would like to bounce on a large ball to stimulate my vestibular nervous system. I was receptive, although I thought she said "bounce" as in "dribble" rather than "bounce on" as in "on top of." Having majored in economics in college, I had a limited science background. I had heard of the central nervous system, but not the "vegetable" nervous system. Even when it was pronounced correctly as the "vestibular" nervous system, I was not familiar with it. Karen explained that it was vaguely related to the inner ear and that by stimulating it, control of my upper body trunk could be improved.

To stimulate the vestibular system, I sat on top of an air-filled ball about three feet in diameter. In this squatting position on top of the ball, I would inch my legs inward to start a gentle rhythm of upward motion and ride the ball like a carousel horse. We did this exercise a half-dozen times, and there was a pronounced improvement in the way I carried my upper body. My posture was improving.

If something as ridiculous as the "vegetable" nervous system and bouncing on a ball could yield such quick and noticeable results, other improvements certainly were possible. Another improvement was that when I would sit in a rocking chair, I could get it rocking using my left leg. I always said that my left leg was paralyzed since I could not move my toes, foot, or ankle, but there was still a connection with my thigh and calves. The wiring was shorted-out, but the connections survived.

While rocking, I would talk to Karen. She was a source of knowledge about the outside world. She wore her braces inside her long pants. I often wanted to ask her to take her pants off so I could see how the braces were fitted, but my inhibitions were not completely gone and I never made the request.

66

A Brace, a Cane

I thought my first meeting with Dr. Garabaldi, the physiatrist who ran the rehabilitation unit, was an accident, but it might have been of his design. One morning after breakfast I was taking a detour on the way back to my room and saw a tall, well-dressed man by the shower area; perhaps his name tag or his commanding presence told me he was my leader.

Since I was fairly young and had a dynamic sling on, I would have been easily recognized without a nurse pointing me out. I stopped, introductions were made, and Dr. Garabaldi and I stumbled through the "how are you" questions. I then asked, "Doctor, please tell me, will I walk?"

With very few preliminary words and with no effort to be evasive, he said, "Fred, please understand it is too early to give you a solid answer. I don't know if you will need a brace or a cane, but I can promise you that you will walk."

I said I would not mind a cane or a brace if they were necessary. I had no idea what type of brace might be appropriate. I thought I would probably need some type of wrap-around bandage to support my knee. And a cane might appear distinguished.

Ambulating

After I spoke with Dr. Garabaldi, I ran into Bruce, the social worker, and I quickly told him that Dr. Garabaldi had confirmed that I would walk. Bruce was not impressed with my good news, and he somberly asked me, "Fred, are you sure he said 'walk' and not 'ambulate'?" Upon the fringe of fear, I replied that the doctor had said "walk"; he thought I might need a brace or a cane, but he said "walk."

Bruce continued to question if I had recalled the conversation correctly, insisting that the best I could hope for was to ambulate. I was not sure what ambulating meant, but I knew that walking had to be preferable to it. As Bruce continued to insist that I might have misinterpreted what the doctor said, I began to have my own self-doubts. Bruce was part of the system, he may have had a unique insider's knowledge. Perhaps by deflating my romantic notion of walking, he was focusing my attention on harsh reality. I was aware enough of harsh reality and resented my balloon being popped.

Bracing

As I attempted to gain my confidence that Dr. Garabaldi really had said that I would walk, I told my physical therapist, Linda, the story, with all the equivocations and qualifiers the doctor had used, and mentioned the canes and braces.

Rather than telling me I had misunderstood the doctor, my physical therapist, Linda, said, "Fred, we have never braced a patient here before, and we are not about to start with you." The fact that a brace was a possible eventuality was lost in the wash. I thought the doctor was the captain of the ship and was frightened that my therapist thought she could set policy at odds with what the doctor might want.

After physical therapy, I was waiting longer than usual for a therapist in occupational therapy. Both Beckie and Karen were on vacation, and being dispirited, I slumped in my chair and cried.

In a moment, a beautiful occupational therapist I had not seen before came over and introduced herself as Nellie and told me that she would be working with me. She asked me why I was crying. I told her about Bruce and ambulating and Linda and braces. Nellie asked me if I would like her to intervene with Linda on my behalf. I replied, "Yes."

Ten minutes later, Nellie came back with Linda. Linda launched into another attack on braces. I felt as if our past discussion about walking had locked us into conflict. Linda seemed to argue that even if I could walk with a brace, the brace was certain to cause long-run problems, that some spasticity would result that might cause me to fall and break my hip, that the brace would weigh so much that I would ultimately abandon it for a wheelchair. (In Linda's defense, years later I did meet a polio victim who had abandoned her heavy, full-length braces in favor of life in a wheelchair.) Linda continued that a brace would not allow the natural return of strength to the leg. (In retrospect, I know I am better off that I was not fitted for a brace.)

Our argument was not yet full blown when Bruce walked up. He reintroduced the notion of ambulating in lieu of walking. My therapist and social worker seemed to be working in concert to confine me to a wheelchair for life. I had seen too many ploys in negotiations to believe that Bruce had just wandered by at an opportune time. The deck was being stacked.

At first I thought that Bruce and Linda were caught up in some institutional imperative to force me to embrace a wheelchair and to forever renounce walking. Many rehabilitation patients in Miami are elderly; Miami has a large elderly population. Thus, their prejudice in favor of wheelchairs might have been reasonable, but I was in my thirties and walking was not an improper goal. And, of course, the bracing issue was a tangential argument that could and should have been avoided. I never wanted a brace, but if it was the price for walking, so be it. One of the hidden costs of this argument was that it reduced my faith in the institution. When I finally checked out, I ignored the sound advice of some personnel I adversely classified as "wheelchairers."

Absentee
Management

I could have better understood the confusion of the hospital program if I had compared it to the corporate structure with which I was most familiar. I was a corporate creature, the man from the home office, and I normally managed responsibilities over the telephone and by mail. I now was caught up in this absentee or corporate-type management, but I did not recognize the clear characteristics.

Although I would have preferred the mythical tall, white-haired, horse-and-buggy doctor who made house calls, I was saddled with an absentee-boss doctor. When I was admitted to the therapy unit, the decision to take me was based on staff reports prepared by competent physical therapists. The boss did not have to examine me personally; he had a well-greased machine and could trust its judgment. Rather than seeing me routinely, Dr. Garabaldi monitored my progress at a weekly staff meeting held on Wednesday afternoons.

This concept was not foreign to me; I had sat behind a desk and done this type of supervision myself. Of course, when it involved some onerous union in some small Indiana town, it was practical modern management. When it was me on the receiving end, it was cold, unfeeling absentee management.

To me, those weekly staff meetings were rather ominous; although their function was never explained to us, it was noticed that some uncooperative patients were asked to leave following the meetings. These exiles and the meetings seemed related.

Since a decision could be made at those staff meetings which affected my well-being, I thought it appropriate to ask Bruce who looked out for my interests at those meetings. He automatically replied, "Well, I do." I was far from certain that my interests could be best served by someone I regarded as a steadfast proponent of the wheelchair school. My union dealings have left me with the deep belief that a person has the right to pick his own representative. It is somewhat beside the point that nothing diabolic befell me as a result of those staff meetings; the possibility was there.

The Alice-in-Wonderland nature of labor relations is nowhere more starkly outlined than in the area of fair representation. A union business agent is required to represent the interest of each member "fairly." The case law that established this principle was in the Supreme Court case *Vala* v. *Sipes*. A company had discharged an employee named Owens, allegedly for his poor health. The employee came up with some medical evidence that he was healthy; grievances were filed. Prior to an arbitration hearing, the union sent Owens to the union doctor to help prepare its case. When their own doctor would not support the claim that Owens was fit for work, the union dumped the grievance. The courts ultimately held that the union did not represent Owens fairly.

As almost every business agent will admit, the union and the company must work together and ordinarily the union will not support bad grievances. That reasonable era came to a close with the *Vala* v. *Sipes* ruling. Unions then started to support any grievance and became overly cautious, operating like doctors fearful of potential malpractice suits.

Although I'm liberal, I never favored the concept of "fair representation," thinking the business agent should be left with the maximum flexibility to trade grievances. That was a milieu with which I was familiar and how I related to the "secret" staff meetings. The meetings seemed pregnant with issues of fair representation. When I asked to be divorced from Sol, it was possible that my request for a new roommate could have hurt Sol's morale. Could or should my interests have been sold short to protect him?

Now, of course, I realize that everyone acted in good faith. "Good faith" is a narrow thread that weaves through the National Labor Relations Act. I used to walk that thread of a tightrope, and I know it was just like dancing in the air.

Certainly it is unkind to point out and question such farfetched hypothetical issues, but please recall that the stroke patient has a great deal of time to be both critical and hypothetical. A closed-door meeting just added fuel to the fire.

Since the meetings were weekly, the possibility of being ostracized was always close at hand. At least in ancient Athens the meetings at which a citizen could be expelled from the city were held yearly. Whatever my misgivings, I felt the meetings allowed the doctor to practice absentee medicine.

Goals and
Group Meetings

At a group meeting Bruce once asked us what our goals were for therapy. I responded that mine was to be made whole. I continued to maintain that strong public posture, but by the middle of summer I had reduced my expectations to, "I will walk by Christmas." I did not have any rigid time line in mind when I picked Christmas.

Christmas is a sentimental holiday, but it *is* also a date certain. I had studied enough economics to realize that you do not put a prediction and a date on the same piece of paper, yet I felt so strongly about this goal of walking by Christmas that I told Judy and also mentioned it in a letter to my parents. I was still afraid to appear too confident and added as a caveat the Robert Browning insight that "a man's reach should exceed his grasp or what's a heaven for?"

Although walking might be considered miracle enough, I was aware that I had significantly lowered my expectations when I said "walking by Christmas" in lieu of "being made whole." That is a significant concession. I was no longer negotiating with God but with my own spirit. And I was afraid to expose too much of my soul to the light.

My soul-baring or concealing was done at a group meeting all patients had to attend. The tables were pushed against the walls of the day room. The patients lined up as best they could in front of Bruce. There would be an undercurrent of tension as we were all asked to introduce ourselves. I believe the aphasic patients benefited from the forced performances. Some of the other stroke victims seemed as tense at being in public forum as did the aphasic ones.

The meeting where I announced that my goal was to be made whole soon got out of hand. A number of patients complained about the food, the impersonality of the program, and the strictly regimented routines. One of the complaints that espe-cially moved Judy was set forth by a kind-looking gray-haired woman who bemoaned the fact that she could not have her tea in the morning. She was accustomed to being dressed before breakfast, and she resented the hurried confusion of our morning schedule. She wanted to get an early start, and she had asked permission to make tea in the morning, but permission had been denied (no doubt a case of a prohibited electrical appliance). I do not know how accurately the lady described her problem, but the story had a ring of truth to it. Of course, an alarm clock and a tea pot could have been excellent tools to prompt some subtle ther-apy. This woman's wish to make tea would have been a good beginning in teaching her how to care for herself again.

However, the staff response to all of the above was that Bay View was not a luxury hotel and that if we did not like the pro-gram, we could go elsewhere. This infuriated me. I retorted that such attitudes were typical of the arrogance that sparked the move toward socialized medicine.

Nathan

Being concerned that I might leap from the frying pan into the fire, I was cautious when I divorced Sol. My new roommate, Nathan Fine, was an elderly man at least seventy-five years old.

The vast difference in our ages might have caused strain, but did not, for I came to love this frail old man. He had a unique courage and grace. Nathan was a Polish Jew who had survived the death camps. The tattooed numbers on his forearm were a beacon at night. When Nathan sat up in bed, he wrapped himself in the bed sheet. The sheet was hood-like over his head and shoulders and took on the appearance of a prayer shawl. With his good arm, Nathan would hold his bad arm out; the concentration camp number seemed luminous. The effect was surrealistic, Chagall-like. As Nathan held his arms out he would make a sweeping gesture with them and tell me, "Fred, God did not let me live for this."

In therapeutic medicine it is all too easy to lose sight of the beautiful dignity of the affirmation of life this man was making. The general line of thought, "I lived through World War II so what could happen to me now," might be thought of as a form of denial of his condition. However, when Nathan would sigh that God did not let him live for this, he was reaffirming a deep belief that he would persevere. Although buffeted by the worst of fates, this old man had a belief in his God and his religion.

At night when I was not negotiating for a shower, Nathan and I would roam the hallways in our wheelchairs. Our jaunts were fairly lengthy. We were two chariots, pulled by our legs instead of horses. The nurses, perhaps pleased to see us active, relented on their prohibitions about leaving the floor. Our jaunts soon took on a ritual importance, and we spoke of them as "running the halls."

A Weekend Home

The general routine of physical therapy exercises was conducted on Saturdays by a special weekend crew of therapists. Although the weekend staff was necessitated by personnel needs, I thought the break from the regular therapists was a welcome relief. Seeing us only once a week, the weekend crew seemed more mindful or willing to comment on the almost imperceptible improvements we were making.

We were encouraged to get a pass to spend the "weekend" at home. The policy of the rehabilitation unit failed to take into account that the weekend actually started on Saturday morning after therapy and ended Saturday night. We were allowed home after therapy on Saturday morning but were expected back the same evening; no overnight stays were allowed. This was a very short weekend, indeed. The hospital justified this policy of fractured weekends by faulting the insurance company regulations, the argument being that if we were capable of spending the night at home, we were capable of being outpatients.

Although no doubt grounded in reality, I thought this was a rather lame excuse. Even if one were to assume that I was capable of being an outpatient, what of the highly vaunted "dorm effect"?

My first weekend home was eventful for both Judy and me. I had been telling Judy for months how well my occupational therapy was going and that I was going to be independent. My first weekend at home was going to allow her to evaluate how independent I was or was not.

I had been in one hospital or another for months and considered the one-day Saturday pass a well-earned vacation. In spite of the positive personality changes I had undergone, I found it very easy to slip back into my prior role as the dictatorial husband

and asked Judy to wait on me hand and foot. Why be independent when you can have a wife-slave?

The straw that broke the camel's back was trivial; it came when I asked Judy to get me some fresh clothes after I had taken a nap. Although I was ready to demonstrate my dressing skills, I had failed to lay out a clean set of clothes before my nap. Judy broke down in tears and asked me what had become of all the skills for independent living I was supposed to have learned. She was reluctant to attack me as strongly as I deserved because we just had some fine sexual relations.

With the death of my sexual inhibitions, I was a more free and spontaneous lover. This wonderful change was coupled with some practical physical realities that forced me to be a better partner. The practical physical reality we had to cope with was that since my left side was paralyzed, I could not plop over Judy in the traditional missionary manner; I had to entice her to come to me. Our sex now had a good deal of give and take rather than a one-sided domination. My physical limitations had turned our lovemaking into a true partnership.

A Setback

My therapy seemed to be progressing well on an uphill path until one morning I suffered an unexpected reverse while in therapy— I had my first seizure. The day started with some exercises with Linda. She was working on helping me to get my toes to uncurl. This was fairly painful, and I welcomed a chance to work on the parallel bars, even when Linda made it clear I was not to try to walk.

I parked at the beginning of the parallel bars and stood while Linda strapped a wide canvas belt around my waist so she could grab me if I fell. I shuffled forward a few feet and we began to exercise. The object was to encourage me to shift weight to the left side of my body. I then detected a sharp taste of spearmint in my mouth and my muscles seemed to go limp. Linda suddenly yelled, "Fred's going to fall. Help me!"

I felt weak and thought that I was going to fall. Rather than toppling forward or backward, however, I more or less just slumped to the floor. I thought rather unkindly that if I was to fall, I was glad it was while I was working with Linda. She would have to write up the incident report.

When I was on the floor, Linda told me not to worry, that I was not having a stroke, only a seizure. I had thought that I had simply fallen down. I was fully conscious, and it had not occurred to me I might be having another stroke. I was taken back to the ward I had been in when I was first admitted to the hospital. I was going to be stabilized.

The seizure weighed heavily on me. With parts of my brain dead it was possible for me to accept that my brain would not work too well. The seizure, rather than stemming from a partic- ular part of the brain, represented my entire brain being in rebel- lion. It was bad enough that my brain did not work; now it had to throw tantrums. On the positive side, if medical science could not cure my seizures, it could at least help control them with medication. I started taking phenobarbital and Dilantin twice a day.

The sharp spearmint taste I had noticed before the seizure was thought to be an aura, an early warning sign that a seizure was imminent. This was a good arrangement. If the medicine failed, I would have some warning before the next seizure. Of course, I failed to take into account that I chewed a great deal of spearmint gum.

Although future seizures were possible, the medicine seemed a perfect remedy, but it was quite potent. My occupational therapy had been fairly intense prior to the seizure; there was a definite thrust to prepare me to leave the hospital. Beckie and I had been working on my wheelchair skills on carpet. Shag carpet will slow down a wheelchair, but I had built up my endurance to an acceptable level. I found that after taking the medicine for my seizures, my endurance was lessened. I was weaker. This marginal loss of strength might appear to be of no great importance, but my strength had been reduced to such a low level that I feared the diminution of any of my strength. When you haven't got much to lose, anything—no matter how minor—was important. The drugs did wonders, but I was paying more than a small price to be free of seizures.

In the beginning chapters of this book, I was more than willing to castigate the medical profession for not warning me that I might have time and space disorientation. Judy felt very strongly that I should have been warned also about the possibility of seizures, though I'm not sure that I would agree with her on this point.

Winding Down

There seemed to be a general consensus that I was ready to leave the program, and the hospital, and go home. Before I went home, I wanted to walk. One morning when I saw Dr. Garabaldi in occupational therapy, I immediately wheeled over to him and demanded that he have the therapists teach me how to walk before I was released.

The doctor asked me if I could walk. I firmly replied, "Of course."

The doctor challenged me by telling me to go ahead and walk. I was befuddled by his response. The parallel bars were in the physical therapy gym next door, and I was not sure what to do. I said, "I can walk with a cane."

The doctor looked around for a cane but none was in sight. He said, "Take my hand. It will be your cane." I held Dr. Garabaldi's hand and took about ten steps. I thought I had done just great and with sheepish grin I said, "See, I can walk. I just need a cane."

The doctor replied, "My arm is not a cane."

"What's the difference?" I asked.

He replied, "My arm lent you balance, a cane will not."

Beckie explained to me that there were other therapists who could work with me as an outpatient, and they would help me with walking. She said, "Fred, walking is between you and God. No one can teach you to walk. If you can, you can, but these other people can help you to walk better."

Although I was anxious to get on with my life, I still relished the warm security the hospital offered. All of my therapists had been friendly, but I found it even easier to talk with them after my discharge was in the works. I think that my therapy treatment was very much an adversarial relationship. With union business agents, I had been used to being locked into combat over the table; after the war is over, a deep calm may set in, and it may turn out that strong bonds had been forged. Whether or not I had been at war with my therapists, I found myself enjoying a new and closer relationship with them.

I learned a good lesson from Karen, the girl who had polio and wore braces. I mentioned to her that I had been in a new shopping center in my wheelchair, and I had almost been trampled by Christmas shoppers. She gave me a knowing smile and said that she kept a wheelchair in the trunk of her car and always used it during the holiday season. I was surprised that Karen would ever use a chair since she could walk with the aid of braces and Canadian canes. She patiently explained to me that being in a chair was less tiring, and it freed up her hands.

I was scheduled to leave the hospital on Wednesday. A wheelchair had been ordered and things were well in hand, except on the Thursday of my last full week, Judy and I decided we could not wait another weekend. So, I requested my release the next day.

Most of my chances for tender good-byes with my therapists were lost with the rushed release. A wheelchair was scraped up; it was a bit plush with its pneumatic bicycle-type tires. I thought I was just going home and that I would resume a normal life immediately. Bruce, the social worker, rather wisely counseled me that I was not yet ready to return to work. Although he was right, I would not heed his advice because I thought he was a leading proponent of the wheelchair school.

Judy picked me up at three o'clock on Friday afternoon to take me home. I jubilantly wheeled out, but I did not "burn my chair" in the parking lot.

On that first day out of the hospital, the signs were not at all auspicious. It was obvious on the drive home that Judy wanted to tell me something; she was reluctant to start. As we got closer to home, she could no longer delay, and she told me that at the beginning of the week a neighborhood gang had a rumble near our house. Our home had been broken into, and my collection of antique firearms had been stolen.

It ultimately turned out that my gun collection, rather than being stolen, had been hidden where Judy could not find it. The antique guns had been manufactured by my great-grandfather, Samuel Watson Johnson. Although they have some real financial value, they have great sentimental value to me, and Judy was reluctant to tell me of their apparent loss. As Judy related her tale, I was pleased to realize that these family heirlooms had not really been lost. I had taken them from the closet and hidden them under the bed before my stroke without telling Judy. Although you do not want to burden someone in the hospital with bad news, I had never stopped to think that Judy did not consider that I was up to receiving the bad news. And I thought I was ready to burn up the world! Perhaps I was not as strong emotionally as I had thought.

It seems as if the fates were conspiring to dampen our enthusiasm. Sunday morning when we woke up, we found that one of the pheumatic tires of my wheelchair was flat. The right front tire of our automobile was flat as well. As Judy changed the car tire, the reality of our role reversal was hammered in with each click of the jack.

The first few days at home were spent learning to cope with the fact that our house would not accommodate a wheelchair very well. Certainly when I had come home on the weekend pass I was aware that there were problems with the house. Now these problems could not be ignored. Our house was fairly new; it was built for us four years earlier. Although I invariably told people I was from Miami (I worked there and people know where it is), I, in fact, lived in Miramar, a bedroom suburb of Miami. Although I had a "new" house in a "new" community, the zoning restrictions did not require doors that were at least wheelchair wide.

I could not wheel into the main bathroom. Fortunately, when the house was built Judy and I resisted the then-current architectural rage of a sunken living room and a conversation pit. At least I had a flat, even floor. Although I could not get into the main bathroom, I could use the commode in the half-bath in our bedroom. The large spacious kitchen, designed to appeal to a housewife, had a stove top and a counter that were too high for me. The wall phones were all in the wrong place.

This litany of grief is not here to suggest that a home should be remodeled before the stroke patient comes home. What needed rehabilitation was not the house, but me. With a little mobility, I could cope with most of the architectural barriers. I don't think my therapists truly understood my zeal to walk, especially the ones who had written me off for limited ambulation at best. The ability to take ten steps can break down countless barriers in the home and is worth the effort.

My mother realized the pressure that was on Judy to hold our family together, and she sent us money to buy a microwave oven and a freezer. I thought these appliances were to help me, but now I realize that they were to help Judy.

Judy learned to cook with the microwave; I only used it to

thaw things. At first I had a great deal of fear of fire and liked our electric stove; I now have a decided preference for gas stoves where I can at least see the flame.

Before I left the hospital, the doctors gave Judy the apparently obligatory lecture about preparing me to sit in front of the TV for the rest of my life. Although Judy had the courage to disbelieve, there were some lingering suspicions about my mental state. We both wanted me to be evaluated by a neutral party: a neuro-psychologist.

The testing was simple. I sat in a large easy chair and answered a series of verbal questions and made up stories to fit some pictures on a storyboard. There were a few math problems and a short paragraph to read. I don't understand the mechanics of testing, but it was determined that I had the ability to reason and had strong verbal skills. On the negative side, it was found that my short-term memory was impaired and that I was tone deaf.

I might not be able to read big numbers, and, although impaired, I could read, but I had my marbles. I was rational.

The Social Safety Net

One of the few things that was handled well at my first hospital was my petition for a disability claim with Social Security. A Social Security agent visited me at the hospital and suggested that I apply for disability payments. I was in one of my "I'm not going to be disabled" moods, but the agent patiently and optimistically explained that it took a long time for the paperwork to be completed so it was best to get it into the hopper. In this way, I would be prepared for any eventuality, and if I did not need it, all the better. The agent explained that even if I was granted the financial help, stroke patients can show unexpected improvements, so I could expect to be reviewed periodically.

Judy was concerned that the chance of gaining a disability claim might cause me to hold back in therapy and that it would be a self-fulfilling prophecy. Her fears were groundless, but Judy was drawn into the process.

A ream of forms was left for Judy to fill out, and we began our introduction to the welfare state. Judy had to get a copy of my birth certificate and a social security number for our son, Sam. The Social Security office was always crowded, and Judy had to draw a number much like you do at the meat counter of a crowded grocery store.

I ultimately was awarded a reasonable disability payment based on my income and prior contributions to Social Security. Sam was also given a meager award.

We were on the dole. With that came certain responsibilities, the nature of which were never entirely clear to me. I realized, however, that it was critical to protect this entitlement. Shortly before my release from Bay View, we were flooded with mail praising the Florida Office of Vocational Rehabilitation. It seemed that the government was willing to spend some money to rehabilitate me; no doubt the hope was to get me off the dole.

Although I myself was certainly anxious to be rehabilitated, the government literature seemed intentionally vague as to whether or not I was required to seek the help of the Office of Vocational Rehabilitation. Recalling all of those heavy-handed stories of the government forcing people on welfare to work, I thought it wise to check out the rehabilitation office, if for no other motive than to keep my skirts clean.

I found that funding for the office had been cut back and that I could expect little help. In Florida, and later in Texas, I was to see that the rehabilitation commissions were blue-collar oriented.

In Florida, the commission looked at me somewhat askance because I was a white-collar worker and because I was still employed. Throughout my months of hospital confinement, the company had kept me on the payroll and was anxious for me to return to work. I requested that the rehabilitation commission provide services that would help me keep my job. I wanted to see if I could drive a car, and I wanted to work with a speech pathologist on my writing and general lack of follow-through. I also requested counseling for Judy and myself.

I am reasonably confident that if my wish list of services had been granted, I would have been better able to hold on to my job. Given the commission's lack of money and my white-collar status, nothing was done. An opportunity was lost. We all have our tales of woe and sorrow.

Even if the state vocational rehabilitation folks had little interest in helping me, I still had my group medical coverage. It would help with physical therapy, but not with the psychological problems.

I began attending a nearby sports medicine facility that had been started by a young licensed physical therapist who was realizing his own entrepreneurial dream of having his own place. Although he had a thriving business at some nursing homes, I was to be one of his first customers at his new facility, which was set up in an old post office he had leased from the General Services Administration. The building itself was in poor shape. I worked on a number of machines that were designed to improve my walking. I walked on some struts that provided varying resistance to each leg. The resistance provided by the machine was determined by the amount of pressure I had exerted with the prior step. I sat on a tractor-type seat and wore a seat belt while doing the exercises. My feet were strapped to the struts. The machine would have been a fit ingredient for one of Edgar Allen Poe's horror classics.

The stationary walking was my principal exercise. To round out the routine, there were some conventional exercises to strengthen my right arm. It is necessary to guard against the urge to overexercise the good arm to achieve a Herculean strength in hopes of compensating for the bad arm. Should the left arm ever start to return, it would be bitterly ironic if the strengthened muscles of the right arm tended to overpower the newly awakened left arm.

Work

I get a little uneasy when I talk about work. I guess I'm still hesitant and reluctant to admit the degree of handicap I had or have. I was not aware of or would not accept my limitations.

I lost my job, and I think the worst part is that I did not see it coming.

Of course, if I had been able (wise enough) to see it coming, it would not have happened. High-level corporate labor relations is mostly smoke and is ill-defined, ephemeral, a game of rings. In the midst of chaos, it requires a steady hand. One does not just flow with the current, one must become the stream. The total immersion required is only possible with the active goodwill and support of your co-workers. Although I had long ago earned the goodwill of my fellow employees, when I went back to work I kept eroding away their support.

My principal liability at work was my mental attitude. I was far more concerned with the practical, physical problems I would confront when I went back than with the work itself. Judy and I sneaked into the office on a Saturday morning. We brought grab bars and installed them in the restroom. As a convenience to me, the swinging door on one of the stalls was removed. In my more paranoid moments, I would recall that everything in the restroom was set up to remind my fellow male employees of my troubles. We placed wooden blocks under the legs of my desk to raise it so that my wheelchair would clear it.

Although the restroom was somewhat of a psychological burden, I could handle my workplace physically, aside from my inability to get to the second floor. The worst barriers were the doors. The slab for the front entryway was not quite flush with the sidewalk, and I could not get past the bump and through the front door. I got into the corporate offices by going through the warehouse of a window plant that was adjacent to our offices. I had to manage a heavy fire door that was at best difficult for an able-bodied person to open. Once inside the offices, I was swallowed up in a sea of shag carpet.

I did not come back to work gradually, but rather tried from the start to maintain a regular five-day week schedule. I did not feel any burst of energy due to the medication I was constantly taking to prevent my seizures. I took a two-hour nap before lunch.

There was no pressure on me to maintain a five-day schedule. I worked it primarily to accommodate our transportation needs. Judy could simply drop me off in the morning on her way to work.

My boss commented on this arrangement one day, suggesting that we should get our transportation needs straightened out and decide which job, mine or Judy's, had the greater importance. The kernel of the discussion was that Judy should cut back on her lower-paid work to protect my higher-paying job. My boss is independently wealthy, and I immediately discounted his comment with the rationalization that he did not understand the economic realities of the real world.

Of course, any astute office politician would have seen the straws in the wind. But I did not notice them and never quite grasped their significance until later.

One day, I had a rather trivial letter to sign, and I noted that my original draft of it was paper clipped to the finished letter. I was not in the habit of comparing my drafts to the finished copy, thus there was no reason for the draft to have been retained. Those more astute in the plotting of corporate terminations would realize that the only reason to keep my original draft would be to build "a file."

Such files are made, of course, after the decision to terminate is made; they are not the basis for any decision. If my file were examined, it would show work that was almost indecipherable. Aside from the expected spelling errors, syllables would be left out. I did not maintain margins. It would take me one full morning to write a page. To my credit, I will claim that the material I composed was good.

Aside from my shortcomings in composition, I had also lost my tact. While I was in the hospital, my workload had been carried by my assistant, a capable young woman I had brought up from the ranks. Since I had given her that very important first "break," she was somewhat overly protective of me. Though I wanted to jump right back into the swim of things, my assistant— in an effort to ensure that I did not overly tax myself—was hesitant to turn things over to me. I jumped to the false conclusion that her reasonable concern was a ploy to usurp my authority, and I resisted, causing unnecessary friction in the office.

Certainly my boss was not getting much of a return on the efforts he must have made to keep me on the payroll all those months. As an added burden, I weighed him down with an additional responsibility when I returned to work and told him, "Social Security has a trial work period and if I work beyond it I could lose my disability check. So be sure to dump me if I cannot hack the work."

Angiogram

Shortly after my release from Bay View, I had been scheduled to have an angiogram to determine what had caused my stroke. The test was not run while I was originally in the hospital because the machine was broken.

I had another seizure the weekend before I was scheduled to go in for the angiogram. I was relaxing in a recliner watching TV when I tasted the sharp, mint flavor in my mouth. Although I had experienced many false alarms, I felt certain that this aura was real. I had the recliner fully extended and was concerned that my legs would get caught in the empty space between the footrest and the front of the chair. I tried to sit upright, but I could not get the recliner to fold in. Before I could yell for help the seizure was upon me. Now it was not a foreign experience; it was possible to notice what was going on. Although my entire body shook, it would be an exaggeration to say it convulsed. My left arm, the bad one, jerked around quite frantically, and later the doctor stated that the extreme jerking motion in my arms was the basis for the rather descriptive name of the seizure, which was named for the great American march king. I had suffered a John Philip Sousa seizure.

The timing of the seizure, right when I was scheduled to return to the hospital, was excellent. It turned out that I had misunderstood Dr. Michaels's instructions for taking my medication. I had been taking less medicine that I should have and was under-medicated. If the coincidence of having the seizure when I was scheduled to go into the hospital was an example of good timing, my boss's decision at the same time to force me to take an unpaid medical leave of absence was an example of poor timing.

In spite of the disaster of my termination at work—which,

in fact, this unpaid medical leave was—the angiogram went without a hitch. In an angiogram, a catheter, or a tube, is run through the body. A radioactive trace element, which is visible on an X-ray scan, can be squirted into the carotid artery in the neck to see if the artery is obstructed. Although the procedure can vary, in my case the tube was fed up through the femoral artery of my inner thigh. As the tube is advanced forward, a dye is released so the doctor knows exactly where the tube is going. The dye is iodine-based and has a very unpleasant taste, causing me to have hot flashes. When the tube was fairly far advanced, a series of X-rays of my neck were taken.

As was expected, there was a massive clot in my left carotid artery. A more ominous and unexpected finding was an ulcerated area in my right carotid artery.

For the Best

In affirming that things happen for the best, it is not necessary to compare the new situation "A" with the old situation "B" and determine whether "A" is indeed better than "B." One should look into the new reality "B" for what is good and not be overly concerned with comparative analysis. However, it seems that manifest in any change is a seed that matures into a need for comparison. Thus, from time to time I have looked over my shoulder to see how things were and can now conclude that indeed things did work out for the better.

At first blush, it is difficult to see any good in losing your job, even though subsequent events clearly showed it was for the better. But there were two unexpected developments.

Within a year of my forced leave of absence, the company was purchased in a leverage buy-out by a New York bank investment group. No doubt the New York bankers may have looked upon me with a more jaundiced eye than the previous owners.

Almost concurrent with my company being bought out by the New York bank, the Reagan administration began its ill-fated crackdown on people receiving Social Security disability payments. When I received word that my case was being reviewed, I was not aware of the massive federal dragnet. I thought my review was part of the normal procedure I had been warned about in the beginning.

Although one wants to preserve one's disability benefits, there is a natural aversion to admitting one is disabled. Even though I could not do first-class labor relations work, if the company had carried me for that extra period it is possible that I would have had to do some fancy explaining if Social Security ruled me fit. The new company owners may not have been disposed to carry me anymore and then I would have been out of work with no disability income.

Given that comparative analysis, it would have to be concluded that losing my job at the time I lost it was for the best—plus the fact that it gave us the impetus to go back to Texas. At the time, though, it was difficult to see much good in any facet of the situation.

Go West, Young Man

Perhaps it was panic, but we cast the die and decided to sell our house in Florida and return to Texas. Judy was the keeper of the checkbook and the budget; she realized that we could not hold on to our house. My mathematical skills and concentration were so impaired that I could not even evaluate her financial decision.

With no house and no job, we had nothing to bind us to Miami.

Judy was born and grew up in Austin, Texas, and had a lot of kin there. I had attended St. Edward's University and the University of Texas, both in Austin. Sam was growing up and would be attending college eventually. Austin offered the University of Texas, justly renowned as a football factory, but more important to us, it was also an inexpensive school of excellent scholastic quality.

Having made the decision to move, we felt some pressure to get on with it. A date for the arrival of the moving van was set. Our house was on the market. It was a home purchaser's dream, a true distress sale. We signed the papers the night we left Dade County. The sale netted us enough cash to pay for the move. We had to carry some paper calling for a hundred-dollar-a-month payment from the new owners.

We set out for the West and on the way made an obligatory last stop at Disney World. The trip to Texas was uneventful. I found I now had a tendency to get carsick; a little Dramamine solved that problem.

The Land

As Judy looked to buy a house in Austin, we realized that if we could not hold on to a house in Florida, we could not buy one in Texas. We decided to sink our money into land with the hope of building in the future. We used all our money as the down payment for two acres in Hays County in the Hill Country just outside of Austin.

While Judy was hunting for land, she was looking for a job as well. She had fifteen years of high-level data processing experience, but most of it was for naught because the machinery had changed so much in the last few years. Her skills were there, but her technical knowledge was obsolete.

Her best job opportunity should have been at Southwestern Bell, where she had a decade of service before we were married; however, the company was caught up in the divestiture of AT&T, and a hiring freeze was on. Their best offer was some part-time work with a full-time job down the road. There would be no fringe benefits in the interim. Judy immediately recognized this work on the "if come" proposition as the unlimited probationary period it really was. Although this was distasteful to her, she took the job. Its part-time nature would allow her to ferry me back and forth to therapy.

Therapy in Texas

It was arranged that I would receive therapy at the local public hospital. I was scheduled for speech, occupational and physical therapy. Judy would drop me off at the front door, get my chair out of the trunk, and I would wheel in.

In occupational therapy, my string of beautiful therapists was broken; instead I had a handsome male, Ben, as my therapist. Ben and I primarily worked on my short-term memory and perception.

In physical therapy, I was back in my groove, and I worked with an exceptionally beautiful young woman, April. Although quite varied, my physical therapy with April was designed to get me to put weight on my left leg and to learn to trust that it would support me. The initial exercises usually involved practicing to stand from a sitting position. Although I would still push off with my good arm, after a while there was a discernible improvement in the amount of weight my left leg could handle.

In speech and language rehabilitation, I worked with another fetching female, Lynne Hayes. She was a talented, young graduate student at the Speech and Hearing Center of the University of Texas. Although we would occasionally joke as to whether she would finish her doctoral dissertation before she could teach me to write a book, she beat me by the widest of margins and received her doctorate in short order.

Lynne returned discipline to my life. She insisted that I do some writing every night and that I proofread it. At first, the progress was slow, but before I was aware of it, her charm motivated me to try hard—and the hard work paid dividends.

The Texas Rehabilitation Commission

In spite of my unproductive experiences with the Florida rehabilitation folks, I decided to try the Texas Rehabilitation Commission (TRC). I soon found that it, too, was blue-collar oriented.

I started off on the wrong foot with the commission when
they had me take some "standard" tests. Before the tests in the
morning, I took my breakfast medicine and by mistake my lunch
medicine also. I had a double dose of phenobarbital. I was a little
groggy, but I could not quite put my finger on what was wrong.
The standard test was done with the ubiquitous "shade in the
bubble" on a scantron answer sheet. At the time, I did not realize
that there was a short circuit in my brain between the part that
figures out the answers and the part that directs my fingers to
"shade in the bubbles and make all erasures clearly, please."
Between being doped up and not being able to use the answer
sheet, I took a real dive on my test.

Although Judy realized that it was disastrous for me to do
so abysmally on the test, I was not concerned. I thought it best
that they realize that I had a mental handicap.

At Judy's prompting I asked for a re-testing, but for reasons
that were never entirely clear to me, my request was denied.
Given my low test results it was not surprising that my counselor
was less than enthusiastic when I told him that my long-term
career goal was in some type of personnel work.

After a great number of contortions, I was able to get the
TRC to agree to evaluate me at their rehabilitation center to see
if I could safely drive a car, although I still had a valid Florida

license. A week before I was to go for the evaluation, I was notified that I had to get a Texas "learner's permit." I froze at the thought of another test and did not apply for the permit.

Although the commission should be praised for giving me the opportunity that they did, their last-minute request seemed designed to winnow me from the program and was less than laudatory.

My diagnosis was that both in Florida and Texas the blue-collar bias of the rehabilitation commission made them less than enthusiastic to help me. Certainly some of the cruelest, or most tasteless, jokes I heard in therapy involved what a stroke victim had to do to get help from the TRC. Part of the unfortunate bias against stroke victims, I believe, is in the misconception that they have few employment needs because they are generally elderly retired people with pensions. I have talked to two senior officials of the TRC who have been deceived by this myth.

This is not a scientific treatise, but rather the tale of a personal journey. Thus, I have avoided any effort to back up my views by quoting statistics. As far as I know, there has been no investigation of the employment status of stroke victims, and the subject, if neglected, merits some study and statistical review.

In the prestigious *National Survey of Strokes*, published by the American Heart Association in 1981, the employment status of stroke victims is not examined. However, some inferences might be drawn from the array of statistics in the survey. In 1975–76, 29.65 percent of all stroke victims were under sixty-five. This age group is below the traditional retirement age and could be assumed to have employment needs. The percentage of fatality by age group is:

Age at Onset	Percent Fatality
under 45	23.9
45–54	28.0
65–74	26.1
75–84	31.2

Source: National Survey of Strokes 75 (March/April, 1981). Used by permission of the American Heart Association, Inc.

Young people have a better chance of surviving a stroke. When considering this data, it might be reasonably concluded that the notion, "Stroke victims have few employment needs because they are elderly retired people," is a myth.

Certainly the matter deserves more refined statistical analysis. Any study in this area is apt to overlook the fact that there

98

is a shadow population which has much the same rehabilitation needs as stroke patients—these are persons with head injuries who may be aphasic or hemiplegic. Given my contact with this group, I would not hesitate to assert their average age is much lower than sixty-five and that they have real employment needs.

Thus, the social service agencies that do not supply employment-related rehabilitative services for stroke victims because of this myth are denying these benefits to head-injury victims as well. Again, this is not a scientific treatise, but my narration of a personal journey. A fitting place to pick up my story again was when Judy resolved to quit Southwestern Bell.

The Maid Business

Having resolved to quit the job she did not really have because of its open-ended probationary period, having land payments to make, and having a crippled husband to support, Judy reached out to help an old friend rather than dwell on her problems.

Although it might be thought that Judy would need her own spirits lifted, she resolved to help pick up the spirits of her former roommate, Tracie. Tracie's husband was out of town, so to relieve her loneliness, Judy packed a picnic basket with fruit, bread, and ham, and Judy, Sam, and I were off to visit her.

Tracie was the vice-president of a large think tank for a major software firm in Austin. Tracie's husband was in the marketing department of the parent company. The couple just built their marvelous dream house overlooking Lake Austin. Although they were living in the home, there were countless little last-minute details of construction work that had to be completed. Tracie herself was tied up with her own job and badly needed a ramrod to see that the minor building jobs were completed.

After we finished our picnic feast, Judy cleaned up the kitchen, which generated large amounts of talk about running a house. To get right to the point, Tracie had very soon hired Judy to be her maid, which included a multitude of duties. Judy's hourly rate was based on the pie-in-the-sky promise of Ma Bell. Aside from overseeing the construction work, it turned out that Judy had a real talent for the maid business. In addition to all the cleaning, she could do the shopping and the mending. She also knew how to cater a business party. She was the perfect executive concierge.

Like the proverbial man with a better mousetrap, the world soon beat a path to our doorstep, and Judy had more business than she could handle. She even had to hire assistants.

Although Judy was working full-time, the nature of her work

allowed her to continue to run the family cab, ferrying Sam to school and me to therapy or to the doctor.

In some circumstances the wife working might be thought to be emasculating. I did not have that problem. What emasculated me was that I could not work. We could have scraped by on my disability payments. Judy was working for her own mental satisfaction as well as the money.

I am very active in a number of stroke groups in Austin and know many therapists. From time to time, I will be asked to speak with a stroke victim. To think of this as counseling is overstating the case. I think of it as working with the stroke victim to help acclimate him or her to life post-stroke. All of these stroke activities lend some dignity to the tragedy that befell me. They are my surrogate job.

I hesitate to add the following because my situation is unique. I can speak. I am stable and have a fair amount of mobility, and Austin has a good transit system for the handicapped. Given these four preconditions, I can get out. I am active in local support groups, not so much because of a missionary zeal, but because I know daytime television rots the mind. I know many stroke victims who are more crippled up by their spouses' hovering over them during the day than they were originally crippled by their stroke. If their spouses worked, many of these folks would be better off. Judy's working forced me to reach out into the community and establish my own identity. Again, I must repeat that I added a few preconditions to this recitation. If a person does not have the means to be independent, it is unusually cruel to demand that they be so. If they do have the means, it is crippling *not* to demand they be independent. In short, we should not let our handicaps cripple us.

TIAs

Memorial Day is the anniversary of my stroke. Although I initially suffered from a great deal of time disorientation, it seems as if there is a very accurate clock in my body. Each year near Memorial Day I experience a great number of TIAs.

A TIA is a transient ischemic attack. In my case that is fancy medical jargon for an on and off again numbness in my arm. Although they are a source of concern and curiosity, I recognize them as the harbingers of hell. They stir up a deep-seated fear when they reappear like clockwork with the approach of each Memorial Day.

The more insensitive of you might be thinking, "Fred, it sounds as if this is psychosomatic. It's all in your head."

Of course it is all in my head; that is the point. For some reason, the blood is temporarily unable to reach my head (thus the word "transient" in TIA) and during this interruption some bodily functions may be impaired. In my case, there is a numbness in the fingers of my left hand and in my arm.

The arm is not the only barometer of the TIA; other functions may also be impaired. Judy's Uncle Elmer, a rather spry seventy-four-year-old man, provides an example of how TIAs can go unrecognized. Uncle Elmer was ready to go fishing one day when he fell off the pier while getting into his boat. He was caught between the boat and the pilings of the pier, and he floundered about in a justified panic. When he extricated himself from his predicament, rather than resting for a minute, he took off running up a hill to his lakeside cabin, which was three hundred yards away.

When he got to the cabin, Elmer's wife noticed that his speech was slurred. The joy of the fishing weekend was lost. Elmer decided to drive back to the city, and on the trip home he suffered some disorientation. He had to pull off to the side of the road to rest and re-orient himself.

Although it may have been easy to assume that Elmer's slurred speech and disorientation were tied to his exhaustion from his mishap at the lake, his doctor thought that they were due to a TIA. He had Elmer take an angiogram. His carotid artery was in good shape, but as a precaution a blood thinner was prescribed. As of this writing, Elmer is hale, hearty, and still fishing on the weekends.

Although Elmer's carotid artery is in good shape, mine is not. I have a section that is ulcerated. That one section could be the cause of my TIAs. A piece of plaque could get caught there, and a logjam might be created, causing a temporary decrease in the flow of blood to my brain. Hopefully, the logjam is just temporary and is soon broken up; if not, a clot is formed, and a stroke results rather than a transient ischemic attack.

Naturally, I'm concerned with my TIAs. The rather strange annual cycle is curious, but the fact that they have been transient in the past does not alleviate my fears.

To experience a period of TIAs is to walk through the valley of the shadow of death. Unfortunately, I did not always have the faith of David to sustain me, and I knew fear. The greatest fear was not so much of death as of another stroke. The fear of losing my right side or becoming aphasic was interlaced with an acute awareness of death.

With other stroke victims, I often preach how well we did to live, but with aphasia or the loss of my good right side in the offing, I sometimes have second thoughts. I still want to sing the gospel of life, but fear is a strong enemy.

Rehabilitation

My rehabilitation was going well with the most gentle of prodding. April, in physical therapy, was able to shame me into leaving my wheelchair at home. Judy would drop me off at the front door of the hospital, and I would walk in. Despite my desire to walk, it was not easy to get me to give up the security of the chair. In occupational therapy, Ben drilled me until I could tell time from a clock. When he pressed me to learn my phone number, I would arrogantly reply that I had learned my lessons well and had my phone number written down so I could find it if needed. With a great deal of patience, Ben advanced me to the point where I knew my phone number. Although I resisted the discipline of speech pathology, I could not resist the charm of my clinician; in time, I was able to turn out a page of writing a day. In order to expose me to some deadline pressure, Lynne suggested that I take a short story writing class offered by the city of Austin at the local O. Henry Museum.

I had some creative spark left and did not have much difficulty doing my weekly assignments. My principal difficulty was in getting Judy to find the time to type my papers. I could not understand her justifiable anger at being pressed into this chore after a long day of work.

The University

My short story writing course was a great success; when it was over, Lynne encouraged me to apply for admission to the University of Texas. My motives for wanting to go to the university were mixed. Like many large state universities, it had a number of entering students who needed some remedial education. At the university this service was provided by the Reading and Study Skills Laboratory, termed RASSL.

I wanted to use the RASSL services to learn to read again, so I applied to audit a few courses. I must have filled out the form incorrectly because in short order I received a letter informing me that I had been re-admitted to the Graduate School of Economics. Graduate school? Hell, all I wanted to do was to learn to read again. In the late 1960s I had attended graduate school at the University of Texas, and the computer still recognized my Social Security number and welcomed me back with open arms. I filed the letter away with some glee and was ready to put the matter out of my mind.

This sequence of events happened around the Fourth of July. I soon began to receive mail about fall orientation. I thought this would involve finding the dean's office and getting a tour of the campus.

During the month of August, I slowly realized that I was registered for the fall semester. Desperation and panic set in as September approached. I had not been able to handle my job among friends; how would I survive at this large, impersonal university?

Although I was middle aged and certainly not as alert and spry as the youngsters with whom I would compete, my age gave me a certain perspective that the young underclassmen often did not have. I realized there was someone I could turn to for help.

As with so many other things, the solution to the problem

was in the root of the problem. I was fearful of the large university. The campus was of such great size and diversity that there must be someone there who could help me if I could just reach out. Being unsure as to where to start, I called the office of the dean of students and found that within that office was an orientation program for handicapped and returning students. I spoke with the woman who ran the program. She was sensitive to my apprehension and scheduled me in one of the final orientation groups before the start of the semester. This accommodation was made even though my paperwork was amuck due to the computer continuing to insist that I was a graduate student in the School of Economics. I had my fill of that dismal science years ago. I insisted, the computer notwithstanding, that I was an undergraduate liberal arts major.

Despite the confusion, she patiently counseled me to come to the orientation. Her willingness to extend herself to help a handicapped student was typical of the attitude of all of the staff and instructors I encountered at the University of Texas.

An Amigo

The campus of the University of Texas is large; it is sometimes referred to by the size of the original tract, "the Forty Acres."

Bruce was right, I do not walk; I ambulate. I certainly do not ambulate well enough to handle forty acres. With that in mind, I had previously bought an Amigo, which is a three-wheel electric chair. It looks a great deal like a scooter. The manufacturer claims with some justification that it is "the friendly wheelchair." It will generally elicit a warmer response from strangers than does the typical ominous motorized chair.

With the Amigo, I had the means to get around campus. After my orientation, I knew where to go. It turned out, as one might expect, that if I wanted to be a student I had to take some courses. When I spoke to the clerks in the registrar's office about auditing courses, I was told to go to the accounting department in the School of Business. Although a student at the university is typically required to take twelve hours of work a semester, I pleaded a case with my liberal arts adviser that given my unusual circumstances it was reasonable to let me carry a light load of two courses for a total of six semester hours.

Like most students, my choice of courses was influenced by my interests, by the time of day the course was offered, and by the location of the classroom. I kept my selections within the university's excellent American Studies program, and so was able to get my classes back-to-back in the same room. By happy coincidence, I had the same instructor for both courses, a good-looking English woman. My two courses were "The History of the American Dream" and "The History of American Radicalism."

Having lost the American Dream when I had my stroke, my choice seemed eminently reasonable. I was perhaps influenced by the fact that one of the assigned texts for the course was Horatio

Alger's *Ragged Dick and Mark the Match Boy.* Such books were just my speed. As a child in the backwoods of the Canadian frontier, my mother had learned to read from Alger's books. If my American Dream course could be criticized for lightweight reading material, my other course more than offset that with John Reed's *Ten Days That Shook the World* and Steinbeck's *The Grapes of Wrath.*

It was time for me to see if the remedial education programs could help me with my reading; I had to wrestle with RASSL. Before I could meet with a counselor, I had to take a battery of intelligence tests. There were more scantron-type answer sheets with which I could not quite cope.

When I finally got my counselor, an extremely attractive young blonde woman, I was not surprised to learn that the test results indicated that I needed help. RASSL was set up to deal with a large volume of students and relied heavily upon a canned series of tapes. This was far from the highly personalized attention I had received for months in my sessions in speech and language rehabilitation.

In an attempt to salvage something from our meeting, my counselor told me that many students were able to improve their reading skills by just reading in a quiet place. Although you have no doubt already concluded that I would believe anything told to me by a beautiful young woman, I was infuriated by her advice. Part of my purpose in attending the university had been to avail myself of the services of RASSL; the payoff was to be given some hackneyed advice to read in a quiet place.

Before my stroke, I would often read and watch TV at the same time. I wanted to regain that skill, so I continued to try to read with the TV on, thinking that with practice I could regain my facility. However, the advice of my RASSL counselor continued to nag me, so I tried reading during the peace and quiet of the day when I was at home alone. To my surprise, her advice was sound; with no distractions, I could read more proficiently. I devoured *The Grapes of Wrath* in short order. I took, and continue to take, great pleasure in the fact that I now can read with some of the ease that once was routine. Although there has been a great improvement, I rarely read for pleasure.

With reading under control, I had to confront test taking. Since my handwriting was illegible, I had been concerned that tests would be a problem. As part of the services for handicapped students, the dean's office would provide test-takers who would write the answers dictated to them. I had never cared for dictation. I was not too happy with the results of my dictation and spoke with my instructor. She told me that university instructors are by necessity gifted at reading illegible handwriting. I did my finals in the dean's office, which gave me a quiet place to work and a good table to write on.

The university made every reasonable accommodation to help me as a handicapped student. The student body was quite friendly. At age thirty-eight, I was a little out of place and could be taken for an old graduate student or perhaps a faculty member. My Amigo did not immediately brand me as handicapped. The university has a large campus, and the reaction of many people to my Amigo was, "What a great idea." It was only when they noticed my cane strapped to the steering column that they knew it was a wheelchair and not a clever scooter.

I would be derelict if I did not compare the 1983 students with the ones I knew in the 1960s my first time around. Perhaps it is a sign of my advancing years, but the women seem younger, more sensual. There seemed also to be a more open Christian fever on the campus, which was coupled with a contradictory anti-clerical attitude. Moderate conservatism (Young Republicans vs. John Birch) had emerged as an acceptable belief. There was a heightened awareness of the need to get a job after graduation; art for art's sake seemed out of fashion. There was less tolerance of dissent.

No doubt the students have changed, but I was not transformed into a good student. The first semester I earned a pair of C's in my two history courses. During the following semester, I received a D in a rather difficult upper-division course in cultural anthropology. Although not earth-shattering, my grades were adequate. My whole purpose in returning to school, aside from RASSL, was to be in a safe environment in which I could get on my feet again.

I have worked with a stroke victim who has an excellent executive background here in Austin. He had no immediate job prospects, and I strongly recommended that he attend the university when he left the local rehabilitation unit. It is an excellent place at which to become reacquainted with the "real world." I have spoken with vocational counselors at the Texas Rehabilitation Commission who cautioned that returning to school might be viewed as running away or as a form of denial. Perhaps there is a grain of truth in that, but I have my doubts. I always admitted that I was a dilettante even though I was in a degree program. My goals at the university were to improve my reading skills and to be independent for eight hours a day.

Judy's Fortunes

The maid business is a hard life; Judy longed for some more traditional work with benefits such as health insurance and paid vacation. I was now fairly stable and independent at home so that she did not need to work an irregular schedule to tend to me.

Judy found some work at Tracie's company. Later, at an office Christmas party, Tracie jested to the chairman of the board of the company that she had made the ultimate sacrifice. She had given up a great maid so the company could have a great employee.

Judy did well at her new job. Within a year she had been made office manager of the Austin office. Many of her alleged obsolete machine skills stood her in good stead. Judy is an excellent machine person; although there are no longer tab operators, a good tab operator can learn to operate a high-speed laser printer in short order. Her natural aptitude for personnel management had been sharply honed after years of managing me, and few data processing employees or programmers could be as cranky as I could be.

As Judy prospered at work, we did well in our finances. We sold the land we originally bought when we came to Texas. In that three years, Judy had tripled our money. With that tidy sum, Judy bought good stocks in the stock market. She has gone from maid, to manager, to financier. With all of those changes she has continued to be a good mother and a good wife. How blessed I have been.

A Stroke of Luck

The president of the Austin Stroke Club gave me a copy of *A Stroke of Luck*, which is a newsletter written by stroke victims for other stroke victims. It is edited and published by Helen Wulf, an aphasic. She is also the author of the book *Aphasia, My World Alone* (also published by Wayne State University Press).

The newsletter had been started with the help of Josephine Simonson, a prominent speech pathologist. The original mailing list, which leaned heavily upon a list of members of the Southwestern Aphasiology Society, mushroomed. As the paper gained wider distribution among stroke victims, its circulation grew from 250 in January 1984 to 2,500 in January 1989.

I was stunned by the stark beauty and power of *A Stroke of Luck*. The writing of its aphasic contributors was truly the speech of the speechless. It echoed a voice crying from the wilderness. I wrote Helen Wulf to volunteer to write a column for the newsletter. She asked me to send in some material. I originally intended to title my column "Twice Blessed," with the thought that since I had not died from the stroke and I did not have aphasia, I was twice blessed. Although I feel she was overly sensitive to the matter, Judy thought the title denigrated aphasics. I valued Judy's judgment and decided to use "God Could Have Written Me a Letter." My first column was based largely upon the first chapter of this book. Most of the volunteer staff of the paper is aphasic and they have difficulty with correspondence. With my typewriter I'm a prolific letter writer. While visiting Austin, Helen Wulf and her husband, Hans, stopped by to visit me. Helen asked me to serve on the staff of *A Stroke of Luck* and to help with the correspondence.

A Speech

In the spring of 1984, I had taken part in a panel discussion at a meeting of the Southwestern Aphasiology Society. A year later, I wrote the past president of the society, Josephine Simonson, to suggest that they invite me back to speak.

I was asked to address the spring meeting of the society at the University of Texas Health Science Center in San Antonio. Although when I had volunteered to speak I had suggested that I discuss my experiences with re-learning to type, the program inexplicably listed me under the title "The Aphasic Speaks." Sam was going to be away that Friday with his school choir, so Judy and I intended to make a weekend of it. We drove down to San Antonio that Friday afternoon and had dinner with a woman who had been a bridesmaid at our wedding. After a rather festive evening, we got up at noon and found our way to the Health Science building. During the lunch break we set up for my speech, which was scheduled next. The medical center was beautiful; the lecture hall was plush. There were tiers of desks that unfolded in a semi-circle in front of a fancy podium. Some of the old magic returned, and the speech went well. My speech was as follows:

> The program reads "The Aphasic Speaks." It humbles me to be included with such a brave group.
>
> Before I talk about writing, I would like to tell you about my introduction to speech pathologists. I'm forty years old and I had my stroke three years ago. After my stroke, I noticed something wrong with my speech; I thought I had a stutter or tremor in my voice.
>
> I made my living negotiating union contracts and was very concerned with my speech delivery. I was a right-hemisphere

patient who normally would not see a speech therapist, but I did not know any better and I insisted on seeing a speech therapist. We did the normal round of Kaputaka.

I did not know if I had a speech problem or not. I think my father's explanation was best; he told me that I was speaking more slowly and more deliberately and that this change was an improvement over my old style. This positive affirmation helped me. Then, using her typical wiles, my therapist tricked me into writing.

One day I got to therapy early, or she was late, and there was a yellow legal pad on her desk. I tried some cursive writing. It never occurred to me that I might have a problem. I was just experimenting. My cursive writing was a mess that no one could read. And, of course, my speech therapist happens to walk in, and she begins to point at each squiggle and asks me to read it. I cannot, but I'm not worried—that's what secretaries are for.

And what do white collar executives do for a living? They sit on their duffs and write. When I get back to work, or so I thought, there will be plenty of time to write. Practice should make my writing better, so I was on to more important things like physical therapy and walking.

When I went back to work, things fell apart. It would take me all morning to write one page and then no one could read it. I left out letters, and I did not keep my margins. Even I had to admit that my writing was a mess.

I came to Texas and signed up for speech therapy with Lynne Hayes. This time, I was not worried about any imagined stutter. I wanted to be creative again. Lynne worked the magic that speech pathologists have, and she restored my confidence and motivation. I signed up for a short story course at the O. Henry Museum in Austin and took some classes at the University of Texas. But no one could read my writing.

I had long ago given up on cursive, so I printed rather than wrote in cursive. Still no one could read it. I was secretly ashamed of my printing. I knew the poor person who had to read it would have trouble.

Since I was ashamed of my printing, I would be mad at the people who read what I wrote. It's not too good an idea to be mad at your audience, but I was. If I go to so much trouble to write it, you better read it! There had to be a better way.

I remembered that years before I could type with the hunt-and-peck method. We heard about a one-handed typewriter and tracked one down. The letters on the board are shifted so that you can touch-type with one hand. I did not want to learn to touch-type. The machine was no good for me.

I then held up what appeared to be a typewriter and continued:

I think perhaps we are a little older than we were when we were in school. This is not a typewriter; it is a printer. It has an automatic paper feed so it is no trouble getting paper in with one hand. It has a viewing screen where the letters are held a few minutes before they are printed on the paper. There is a cursor to correct my mistakes. No need to worry about Wite-out. This machine is almost a word processor. Do I type perfect copy with it? No, that was never my goal. I just wanted to produce work that was legible, that people could read. Notice how I can always find an excuse for sloppy work.

Although I'm not promoting a particular brand, this machine is a Brother printer from Sears. It runs about two hundred dollars. It is light and truly portable. Thank God I haven't dropped it yet. I have been working on a book about my experiences with rehabilitative medicine. Perhaps you have read the first chapter recently published in *A Stroke of Luck.* It is called "God Could Have Written Me a Letter."

As I wrote it in my green notebook, I had this secret fear that I might have another stroke and be aphasic. My notebook and the first draft of my book would be lost between the cracks because no one could read them. It would have been such a waste. With my printer I have been able to get enough of my book typed to ensure that it will not be lost.

Of course, the more I typed, the better I got at it. This machine has set me free. Should all stoke victims write a book? Not necessarily, but using *A Stroke of Luck* as a source of addresses, we should write each other.

I correspond with a man in Arizona who I think is ashamed of his writing. This machine could help him.

It is fine and good to say or think, "Fred has done well with his typewriter." Of course, it was only after months of ther-apy that I had the gumption to write at all. Although my therapist, Lynne Hayes, deserves great credit, I think the primary credit should go to you and your profession. For a number of right-hemispheric victims and aphasics, you and your art represent salvation, and, on behalf of those others who could not be here today, I would like to thank you. It must be wonderful to work in a profession where you can help people.

Thank you all for giving and for listening to me; if you have any questions, please feel free to jump in.

A question and answer period then followed. Here are two of the questions and my answers:

Q: What do you think of a word processor like an Apple II?
A: My son has an Apple II, and I must admit that I look forward to graduating to the Apple, but in the beginning I think it would have been too intimidating, and it would have scared me off. This little printer is my training wheel for the more advanced machine.

Q: What are your goals in life?
A: I want to finish my book on stroke therapy and move on to a novel that has a little more sex and violence.

The speech was a hummer; it was well received. I got the first standing ovation of my life. When I used to watch the sea gulls over Biscayne Bay while a patient at Bay View, I though that God would give me my left arm back so I could gesture better and speak more effectively. In San Antonio I found I was speaking better than I ever had in my life.

From that San Antonio speech, I re-learned something that I had forgotten, which is to give a good speech you need both a good subject and a good audience.

My subject matter for this book, a stroke, has been a good one. Thank you, readers of this book, for making it this far with me. You are a great audience. Before winding down, though, I have a few more thoughts.

Reading Revisited

On September 5, 1985, I took a reading evaluation test on an Apple computer. I read 230 words a minute with 100 percent comprehension, which was certainly not too shabby for a person who thought he was doomed to never read again. Yes, I can read now, but not with the ease and grace I once did. Now it is work to read.

I am inclined to believe that my improvement in reading was directly related to my increasing ability to write and to be independent. I hesitate to write this for fear it would encourage medical practitioners to adopt an attitude of "let's wait and see" about reading. Although it might be thought that the wait-and-see attitude is reasonable, I submit that it runs contrary to all of the currents of modern rehabilitative medicine.

At the first hospital, Judy was strongly advised not to bring reading material for fear it might frustrate me, as indeed it did. This attempt to deny me reading material is equivalent to asking me not to move my left arm so I will not know it is paralyzed. There were so many stray magazines and newspapers around the hospital and so much time spent waiting, that I was bound to try and read. As a result, I was reading the worst materials under the worst circumstances. The attitude of "let's not let him read now, it might frustrate him" smacks of denial. Dr. Howard Rusk, the father of modern rehabilitation medicine, has taught that inactivity breeds anxiety. As we saw in the prior chapters, the inactivity about addressing my reading problems did breed anxiety. Since we were barred from competent help (which would normally come from the speech pathologist) we muddled through as best we could.

Reading is not just a mental process, it is also physical. I had some straightforward physical problems to overcome; it was difficult to even hold a hardcover book with one hand. Consequently, I switched to paperback books. Although paperbacks are easier to hold than hardcover books, the paperback solution had one drawback. The quality of print and paper often leaves a good deal to be desired. I had found reading to be much easier with high quality matte-finish white paper that is found in better hardcover books. After years of effort, I have mastered the techniques of leaning back and balancing a hardcover on my breastbone and turning the pages with one hand. If the book is too thick for this method, I break its spine and lay it on my desk using two staplers as weights to hold it open.

Newspapers present unique problems. We have a grand maple dining room table that I co-opt on Saturday mornings, pushing cereal boxes and salt and pepper shakers to one end. Even with such a large flat surface, it is difficult to turn the page of a newspaper. Although the quality of the paper is poor, a newspaper has the virtue that you are not expected to read the whole thing. Reading the whole thing is a battle I often face when I read anything.

I read today in part because, by the grace of God, my stroke did not devastate that part of the brain responsible for reading, and in part because Lynne Hayes taught me to follow through—when I pick up a book, I *must* finish it.

This compulsion to complete tasks can be a curse, for there are some books not worth finishing. Before my stroke I would exercise critical literary judgment and sometimes give up on a book after twenty pages. Because of Lynne's lessons, I am often afraid that my critical judgment is just an excuse to get out of a laborious task. Now I read at least one hundred pages before giving up on a book.

Throughout therapy there was a general emphasis on starting soon and working hard. It was reminiscent of the Civil War general advising his troops, "Be there firstest with the mostest!" That seems like sage advice, thus I question the wisdom of not confronting reading problems because they are apt to upset the patient.

Computer viewing screens have received very negative press for the allegedly adverse effects they have on the eyes. As illustrated by the results of my reading tests, however, I did well reading from a screen.

In spite of all my reading improvements, I have not regained my ability to read or understand multi-digit numbers. Reading still is a continual struggle. Unlike many of my other problems, though, with practice (exercise) it has improved.

Walking, After a Fashion

Perhaps the more precise description of my locomotion might be "ambulating." I retain a strong aversion to that word and describe what I do as "walking, after a fashion."

My reading picked up strength with practice, but my walking has not. Although my balance has improved and I am more sure-footed, I cannot walk any more now than I could a few years ago. I have no endurance. I had erroneously thought that the more I did something the stronger I would get; to build up my endurance I just needed to walk more. Unfortunately, this common-sense principle does not seem to apply after a stroke. The reason seems to be in the misconception that a stroke only hits one side of the body. My left side was affected, but there may have been a residual effect down the middle of my body. My lungs and ability to breath may have been adversely affected by the stroke. If I walk more than a block, I get very short of breath; I am fatigued with the slightest activity.

Judy has not been able to find any compassion for my loss of endurance, and she is quick to remind me, "Use it or lose it!" It is difficult for me to get too enthusiastic about exercise when I do not feel it will work. Although exercise may not work with walking, the continual ranging and manipulation of my left arm has yielded positive results.

Since my walking is not up to par, I often am in public with my electric chair. On occasion, I have been asked to speak to handicapped patients at the Texas Rehabilitation Institute. One night, nearly the entire audience was composed of quadriplegics, who are truly the wheelchair bound. I was ashamed that I had driven in my wheelchair rather than walked in.

After so much effort to walk and given my love-hate relationship with my chair, one might expect I would walk as much as possible. The fatigue has taught me what I never wanted to accept—the chair is just a tool, a friend.

Private Conversation

Although I am not aphasic, my speech in private conversations has been affected by more than the imagined stutter or tremor. When I am engaged in private conversation, I think about what I am going to say. I see the words I am considering saying, and they seem to flow across the back of my optic nerve as if on a ticker tape. I evaluate each word to decide if it is worth the effort to push it through the various channels of my brain so that it will attain verbal expression.

At times I might decide not to make the effort, and an entire unspoken conversation will dance across the ticker tape. Oddly enough, this ticker-tape phenomenon does not affect me when I am engaged in public speaking. I am at a loss to explain this anomaly, but would offer this possible explanation. Ever since the sixth grade I have been engaged in high-caliber, high-pressure public speaking. Those endless hours of debate and negotiations might have formed some special, dedicated pathways in my brain for this type of oration under pressure. If such pathways existed, perhaps the synapses were not snapped by the stroke.

An alternative explanation may be a variation of Parkinson's Law: "Work expands so as to fill the time available for its completion." It is possible that in my private, low-key conversations my thought processes have the time to review the ticker tape. In public speaking, time is not available for such digressions. The explanation is beyond the scope of this book or the expertise of this author, it is in the realm of the competent speech pathologist. Judy maintains that when I'm fatigued by the ticker-tape phenomenon in our private conversations, I will sometimes become aggressive in order to bait her into a fight so that I can downshift to my public-speaking mode of conversation, which requires less thought and energy.

120

Settling Up

I have been thinking all along about how to write this final chapter. Since this has been the story of a large slice of my life, I hate to say, "The End." Perhaps it would be less chilling to say, "In conclusion" or "Upon reflection." A sympathetic editor could help by binding in a few blank pages. It doesn't seem fitting to wind my story down with a dry "In conclusion" or "In retrospect." So, one more story.

Before I came home from the hospital, the Patricia Neal story aired on network television. When it was over, Sam began cursing with the anger of an eleven-year-old, stating, "Mother, it isn't fair, all the shows on television have a happy ending. Why can't our life have a happy ending?"

Judy, with a gentle insight, hugged Sam while saying, "Honey, not to worry; our life is not over. We have yet to live our ending."

Fred K. Johnson currently works as a staff member and featured columnist on *A Stroke of Luck*, a newsletter for stroke survivors. He is the former director of labor relations for Keller Industries, Inc., a Miami-based manufacturing company on the New York Stock Exchange. He holds the B.A. degree from St. Edward's University. Johnson frequently speaks about strokes and rehabilitative medicine, relying upon his own experiences as a stroke survivor. He has addressed the Southwestern Aphasiology Society and speaks to students and professionals interested in rehabilitative medicine. He is active in a number of informal support groups and has served on the American Heart Association Stroke Club Awareness Task Force for Texas.

The manuscript was edited by Anne M. G. Adamus. The book was designed by Elizabeth Hansen. The display face is Futura Extra Bold Condensed. The typeface for the text is Trump. The book is printed on 50-lb. Spring Forge paper and is bound in Joanna Arrestox B-grade cloth.

CPSIA information can be obtained
at www.ICGtesting.com
Printed in the USA
LVHW080915310520
657014LV00006B/30/J